KETO
MEAL PREP

*Tasty Recipes to Improve Your Appearance
and Feel Fit*

MAX LOREN

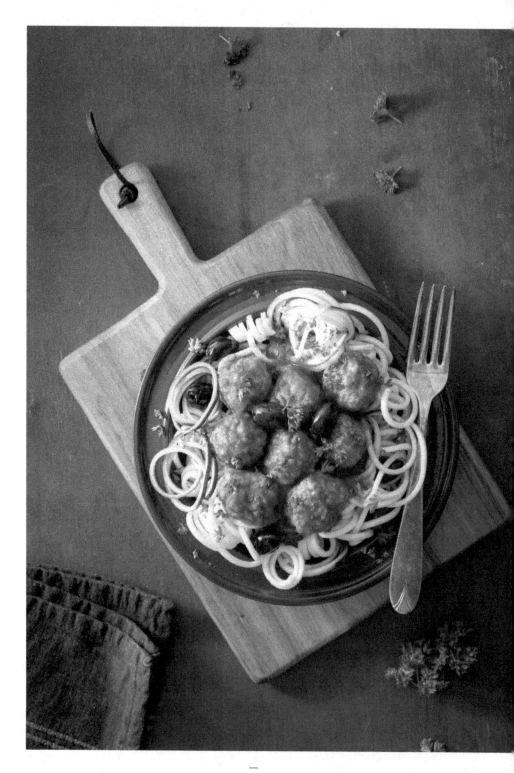

Table of Contents

Sommario

TABLE OF CONTENTS...5

INTRODUCTION...7
  WHAT IS A KETOGENIC DIET?... 7
  DIFFERENT TYPES OF KETOGENIC DIETS 8
  WHAT IS KETOSIS?... 9
  KETOGENIC DIETS CAN HELP YOU LOSE WEIGHT 10
  OTHER HEALTH BENEFITS OF KETO 10
  FOODS TO AVOID.. 12
  FOODS TO EAT 13
  HEALTHY KETO SNACKS 14
  KETO TIPS AND TRICKS 15
  TIPS FOR EATING OUT ON A KETOGENIC DIET........................ 15

BREAKFAST 18
  EGG CASSEROLE.. 19
  FLAXSEED, MAPLE & PUMPKIN MUFFIN 20
  AVOCADO SAUSAGE STACKS 22
  SPINACH-MUSHROOM FRITTATA.. 23
  ITALIAN TOMATO AND CHEESE STUFFED PEPPERS 25
  AVOCADO SAUCED CUCUMBER NOODLES............................. 27
  BROCCOLI AND CAULIFLOWER MASH 29
  SAUSAGE FRITTATA 31
  CHEDDAR & BACON CASSEROLE 32

FISH AND SEAFOOD..33
  COCONUT SHRIMP CURRY... 34
  SLOW COOKED POACHED SALMON 36
  CREAMY KALE SALAD 38
  TROUT CAKES 40
  SLOW COOKED SALMON FILLETS 41
  SHRIMP ALFREDO 42
  HADDOCK CHOWDER 44
  BLACKENED SALMON WITH AVOCADO SALSA 45
  BRAISED SALMON 47
  SEA BASS RAGOUT 48
  ALASKA COD WITH BUTTER GARLIC SAUCE.......................... 49
  COCONUT MUSSELS.. 51
  TUNA CAKES WITH SEEDS 53
  CHIMICHURRI GRILLED SHRIMP 55
  PARMESAN-GARLIC SALMON WITH ASPARAGUS 57

CREAMY HERBED SALMON 59
FENNEL AND TROUT PARCELS 61
SCALLOPS WITH CREAMY BACON SAUCE 63
ALMOND BREADED HOKI 65
TOMATO AND OLIVE TILAPIA FLILLETS 67
CURRIED FISH WITH SUPER GREENS 69

SOUP **71**

CELERY SOUP WITH HAM 72
SAUERKRAUT AND ORGANIC SAUSAGE SOUP 74
CHEESY COCONUT CARROT SOUP 76
CHICKEN GARLIC SOUP 78
BEEF STOCK 80
ITALIAN PORK SAUSAGE AND ZOODLE SOUP 81
LIGHT ZUCCHINI SOUP 83

SNACKS AND APPETIZER **84**

CRAB DIP 85
BAKERY MINI ALMOND MUFFINS 86
CORN DIP 88
CHICKEN WRAPPED PROVOLONE AND PROSCIUTTO 89
MEXICAN DIP 91
CHEESE BISCUITS 92
PARTY SNACK MIX 94

DESSERT **95**

ALMONDS, WALNUTS AND MANGO BOWLS 96
DUMP CAKE 98
EASY MONKEY ROLLS 100
APRICOT SPOON CAKE 101
BERRY MARMALADE 102
RUM BROWNIES 104
PEANUT AND CHOCOLATE BALLS 106

OTHER KETO RECIPES **108**

OMELETTE WITH CABBAGE AND BACON 109
CHICKEN WITH CHEESE 112
STEW WITH SAUSAGE 113
CRAB MEATBALLS AND VEGETABLES 115
BEEF AND SPINACH SALAD 118
BALLS WITH SAUSAGE, MORTADELLA AND ALMONDS 119
TURKEY SOUP WITH GREEN BEANS 121
BROCCOLI WITH SARDINES 122
MOUSSE WITH COFFEE AND CHOCOLATE 124
SRIRACHA SAUCE 126

Introduction

The ketogenic diet, or keto diet, is a low-carbohydrate, high-fat diet that provides many health benefits.Many studies have shown that this type of diet can help you reduce and improve your health.Ketogenic diets may even have benefits against diabetes, cancer, epilepsy, and Alzheimer's disease.

What is a ketogenic diet?

The ketogenic diet is a low carbohydrate, high-fat diet that has many similarities to the Atkins and low carb diets.It involves drastically reducing carbohydrate intake and replacing carbohydrates with fat. This drastic reduction in carbs puts your body into a metabolic state called ketosis.When this occurs, your body is incredibly efficient at burning fat for energy. It also converts fat into ketones within the liver, which can form the energy for the brain.Ketogenic diets can cause major reductions in blood glucose and insulin levels. This, along with the increase in ketones, has health benefits.

Different types of ketogenic diets

There are several versions of the ketogenic diet, including:

The standard ketogenic diet (SKD): This is often a low carb, moderate protein, and high-fat diet. It typically contains 70% fat, 20% protein, and only 10% carbs (9Trusted Source).

The cyclical ketogenic diet (CKD): This diet involves periods of upper carb refeeds, like 5 ketogenic days followed by 2 high carb days.

The targeted ketogenic diet (TKD): This diet allows you to feature carbs around workouts.

High protein ketogenic diet: this is often almost like a typical ketogenic diet, but includes more protein. The ratio is usually 60% fat, 35% protein, and 5% carbs.

However, only the quality and high protein ketogenic diets are studied extensively. Cyclical or targeted ketogenic diets are more advanced methods and are primarily employed by bodybuilders or athletes.

What is ketosis?

Ketosis may be a metabolic state during which your body uses fat for fuel rather than carbs.

It occurs once you significantly reduce your consumption of carbohydrates, limiting your body's supply of glucose (sugar), which is that the main source of energy for the cells.

Following a ketogenic diet is that the best thanks to entering ketosis. Generally, this involves limiting carb consumption to around 20 to 50 grams per day and filling abreast of fats, like meat, fish, eggs, nuts, and healthy oils

It's also important to moderate your protein consumption, this is often because protein can be converted into glucose if consumed in high amounts, which can slow your transition into ketosis

Practicing intermittent fasting could also assist you to enter ketosis faster. There are many various sorts of intermittent fasting, but the foremost common method involves limiting food intake to around 8 hours per day and fasting for the remaining 16 hours

Blood, urine, and breath tests are available, which may help determine whether you've entered ketosis by measuring the number of ketones produced by your body.

Certain symptoms can also indicate that you've entered ketosis, including increased thirst, dry mouth, frequent urination, and decreased hunger or appetite

Ketogenic diets can help you lose weight

A ketogenic diet is also an effective solution for losing weight and decreasing risk factors for disease.

Research has shown that the ketogenic diet can be very effective for weight loss as a low-fat diet.

What's more, the diet is so rich that you can lose weight without needing to count calories or track your food intake.

An analysis of 13 studies revealed that following a low-carb ketogenic diet was slightly superior for long-term weight loss compared to a low-fat diet.

It also led to a reduction in diastolic blood pressure and triglyceride levels.

Other health benefits of keto

- The ketogenic diet originated as a method of treating neurological diseases such as epilepsy.
- Studies have now shown that this diet may have benefits for a wide variety of different health conditions:

- Heart disease. The ketogenic diet can help improve risk factors such as body fat, HDL (good) cholesterol levels, blood pressure, and blood sugar.

- Cancer. Diet is currently being explored as an adjunct treatment for cancer because it may help slow tumor growth.

- Alzheimer's disease. The keto diet may help reduce the symptoms of Alzheimer's disease and slow its progression.

- Epilepsy. Research has shown that the ketogenic diet can cause significant reductions in seizures in epileptic children.

- Parkinson's disease. Although more research is needed, one study found that the diet helped improve symptoms of Parkinson's disease.

- Polycystic ovary syndrome. The ketogenic diet may help reduce insulin levels, which may play a key role in polycystic ovary syndrome.

- Brain injury. Some research suggests that the diet may improve the outcomes of traumatic brain injuries.

However, keep in mind that research in many of these areas is far from conclusive.

Foods to avoid

Any food high in carbohydrates should be reduced.
Here is a list of foods that should be reduced or eliminated on a ketogenic diet:

sugary foods: soda, juice, smoothies, cake, ice cream, candy, etc.

grains or starches: wheat products, rice, pasta, cereals, etc.

fruits: all fruits, except small portions of berries such as strawberries

beans or legumes: peas, beans, lentils, chickpeas, etc.

root and tuber vegetables: potatoes, sweet potatoes, carrots, parsnips, etc.

low-fat or diet products: low-fat mayonnaise, salad dressings, and condiments

some condiments or sauces: barbecue sauce, honey mustard, teriyaki sauce, ketchup, etc.

unhealthy fats: processed vegetable oils, mayonnaise, etc.

alcohol: beer, wine, liquor, mixed drinks

sugar-free diet foods: sugar-free candy, syrups, puddings, sweeteners, desserts, etc.

Foods to eat

You should focus most of your meals on these foods:

meat: red meat, steak, ham, sausage, bacon, chicken, and turkey

fatty fish: salmon, trout, tuna, and mackerel

eggs: whole pastured eggs or omega-3s

butter and cream: grass-fed butter and heavy cream

cheese: non-processed cheeses such as cheddar, goat, cream, blue, or mozzarella cheese

nuts and seeds: almonds, walnuts, flaxseeds, pumpkin seeds, chia seeds, etc.

healthy oils: extra virgin olive oil, coconut oil, and avocado oil

avocado: whole avocado or freshly made guacamole

low carb vegetables: green vegetables, tomatoes, onions, peppers, etc.

seasonings: salt, pepper, herbs, and spices

It's best to base your diet primarily on whole, single-ingredient foods. Here's a list of 44 healthy low-carb foods.

Healthy keto snacks

In case you get the urge to eat between meals, here are some healthy, keto-approved snacks:

fatty meat or fish

cheese

a handful of nuts or seeds

keto sushi bites

olives

one or two hard-boiled or deviled eggs

keto-friendly snack bars

90 percent dark chocolate

whole Greek yogurt mixed with nut butter and cocoa powder

peppers and guacamole

strawberries and plain cottage cheese

celery with salsa and guacamole

beef jerky

smaller portions of leftover meals

fat bombs

Keto tips and tricks

Although starting the ketogenic diet can be difficult, there are several tips and tricks you can use to make it easier.

Start by familiarizing yourself with food labels and checking the grams of fat, carbohydrates, and fiber to determine how your favorite foods can fit into your diet.

Planning your meals can also be beneficial and can help you save extra time during the week.

Tips for eating out on a ketogenic diet

Many restaurant meals can be made keto-friendly.

Most restaurants offer some type of meat or fish dish. Order this food and replace any high-carb food with extra vegetables.

Egg meals are also a good option, such as an omelet or eggs and bacon.

Another favorite meal is burgers without a bun. You could also replace the fries with veggies. Add extra avocado, cheese, bacon, or eggs.

In Mexican restaurants, you can enjoy any type of meat with extra cheese, guacamole, salsa, and sour cream.

For dessert, ask for a tray of mixed cheeses or berries with cream.

At least, in the beginning, it's crucial to eat until you're full and avoid cutting calories too much. Usually, a ketogenic diet involves weight loss without intentional calorie restriction.

In this Keto cookbook, you can organize your Keto diet with the different dishes you'll find for meals throughout the day. Enjoy!

Breakfast

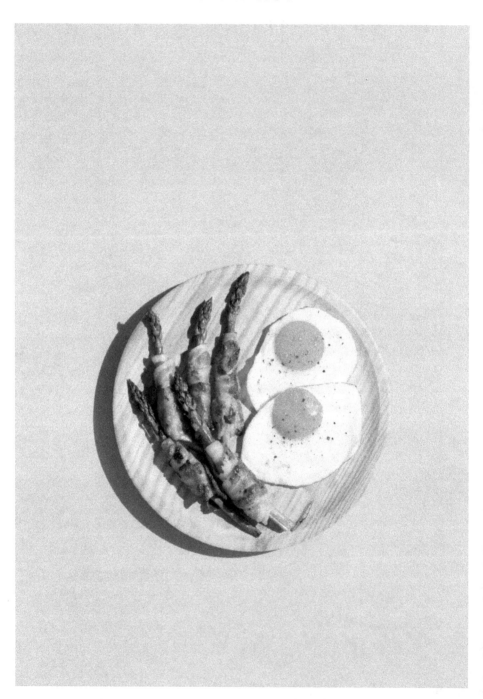

Egg Casserole

Preparation time: 10 minutes
Cooking time: 6 hours
Servings: 4

Ingredients:
¾ cup milk
½ teaspoon salt
8 large eggs
½ teaspoon dry mustard
¼ teaspoon black pepper
4 cups hash brown potatoes, partially thawed
½ cup green bell pepper, chopped
4 green onions, chopped
12 ounces ham, diced
½ cup red bell pepper, chopped
1½ cups cheddar cheese, shredded

Directions:
Whisk together eggs, dry mustard, milk, salt and black pepper in a large bowl. Grease the crockpot and put 1/3 of the hash brown potatoes, salt and black pepper. Layer with 1/3 of the diced ham, red bell peppers, green bell peppers, green onions and cheese. Repeat the layers twice, ending with the cheese and top with the egg mixture. Cover and cook on LOW for about 6 hours. Serve this delicious casserole for breakfast.

Nutrition:
calories 453, fat 26g, carbohydrates 32.6g

Flaxseed, Maple & Pumpkin Muffin

Preparation Time: 10 minutes
Cooking Time: 30 minutes
Servings: 6

Ingredients:
1 tbsp. cinnamon
1 cup pure pumpkin puree
tbsp. pumpkin pie spice
tbsp. coconut oil
1 egg
1/2 tbsp. baking powder
1/2 tsp. salt
1/2 tsp. apple cider vinegar
1/2 tsp. vanilla extract
1/3 cup erythritol
1 1/4 cup flaxseeds (ground)
1/4 cup Maple Syrup

Directions:
Line ten muffin tins with ten muffin liners and preheat oven to 350oF.
All the ingredients must be blended until smooth and creamy, around 5 minutes.
Evenly divide batter into prepared muffin tins.
Pop in the oven and let it bake for 20 minutes or until tops are lightly browned.
Let it cool. Evenly divide into suggested servings and place in meal prep containers.

Nutrition:
calories 241, fat 11.3g, fiber 15.9g, carbohydrates 3.1 g, protein 8.9g

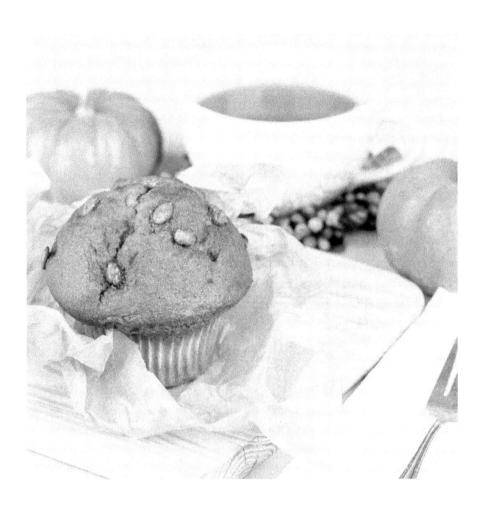

Avocado Sausage Stacks

Preparation time: 5 minutes
Cooking time: 15 minutes
Servings: 6

Ingredients:
6 Italian sausage patties
4 tablespoons olive oil
2 ripe avocados, pitted
2 teaspoons fresh lime juice
Salt and black pepper to taste
6 fresh eggs
Red pepper flakes to garnish

Directions:
In a skillet, warm the oil over medium heat and fry the sausage patties about 8 minutes until lightly browned and firm. Remove the patties to a plate.
Spoon the avocado into a bowl, mash with the lime juice, and season with salt and black pepper. Spread the mash on the sausages.
Boil 3 cups of water in a wide pan over high heat, and reduce to simmer (don't boil).
Crack each egg into a small bowl and gently put the egg into the simmering water; poach for 2 to 3 minutes. Use a perforated spoon to remove from the water on a paper towel to dry. Repeat with the other 5 eggs. Top each stack with a poached egg, sprinkle with chili flakes, salt, black pepper, and chives. Serve with turnip wedges.

Nutrition:
calories 388, fat 22.9g, protein 16.1g, carbs 9.6g, net carbs 5.1g, fiber 4.5g

Spinach-Mushroom Frittata

Preparation Time: 10 minutes
Cooking Time: 15 minutes
Servings: 6

Ingredients:
2 tablespoons olive oil
1 cup sliced fresh mushrooms
1 cup shredded spinach
6 bacon slices, cooked and chopped
10 large eggs, beaten
1/2 cup crumbled goat cheese
Sea salt
Freshly ground black pepper

Directions:
Preheat the oven to 350°F.
Heat olive oil and sauté the mushrooms until lightly browned about 3 minutes.
Add the spinach and bacon and sauté until the greens are wilted about 1 minute.
Add the eggs and cook, lifting the edges of the frittata with a spatula so uncooked egg flow underneath, for 3 to 4 minutes.
Sprinkle with crumbled goat cheese and season lightly with salt and pepper.
Bake until set and lightly browned, about 15 minutes.
Remove the frittata from the oven, and let it stand for 5 minutes.
Cut into six wedges and serve immediately.

Nutrition:
calories 312, fat 6.8g, fiber 5.1g, carbohydrates 3.1 g, protein 10.5g

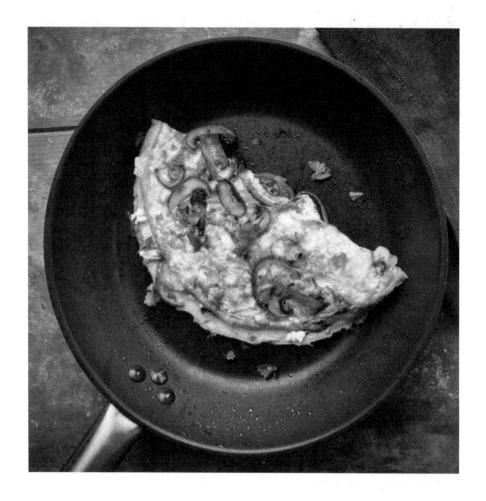

Italian Tomato and Cheese Stuffed Peppers

Preparation time: 15 minutes
Cooking time: 10 minutes
Servings: 2

Ingredients:
1 tablespoon canola oil
1 garlic clove, pressed
½ cup celery, finely chopped
½ Spanish onion, finely chopped
4 ounces (113 g) pork, ground
Sea salt, to taste
teaspoon Italian seasoning mix
sweet Italian peppers, deveined and halved
1 large-sized Roma tomato, puréed
½ cup Cheddar cheese, grated

Directions:
Heat the canola oil in a sauté pan over medium-high heat. Now, sauté the garlic, celery, and onion until they have softened.
Stir in the ground pork and cook for a further 3 minutes or until no longer pink. Sprinkle with salt and Italian seasoning mix. Divide the filling mixture between the pepper halves.
Add the puréed tomato to a lightly greased baking dish; place the stuffed peppers in the baking dish.
Bake in the preheated oven at 390°F (199°C) for 20 minutes. Top with the Cheddar cheese and bake an additional 4 to 6 minutes or until the cheese is bubbling. Serve warm and enjoy!

Nutrition:
calories 312, fat 21.4g, protein 20.2g, carbs 5.7g, net carbs 3.8g, fiber 1.9g

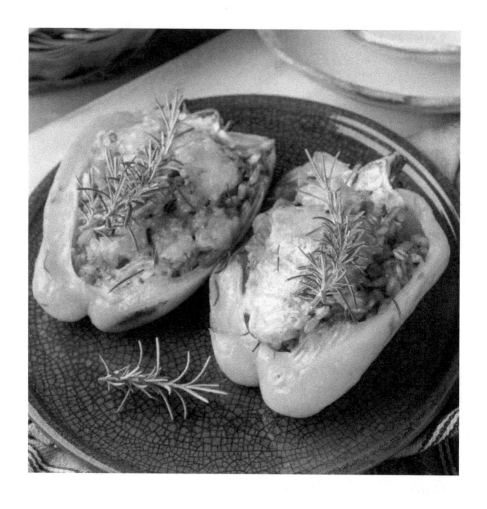

Avocado Sauced Cucumber Noodles

Preparation time: 15 minutes
Cooking time: 0 minutes
Servings: 2

Ingredients:

½ teaspoon sea salt

1 cucumber, spiralized

1 California avocado, pitted, peeled and mashed

1 tablespoon olive oil

½ teaspoon garlic powder

½ teaspoon paprika

1 tablespoon fresh lime juice

Directions:

Toss your cucumber with salt and let it sit for 30 minutes; discard the excess water and pat dry.

In a mixing bowl, thoroughly combine the avocado with the olive oil, garlic powder, paprika, and lime juice.

Add the sauce to the cucumber noodles and serve immediately. Bon appétit!

Nutrition:

calories 195, fat 17.2g, protein 2.6g, carbs 7.6g, net carbs 3.0g, fiber 4.6g

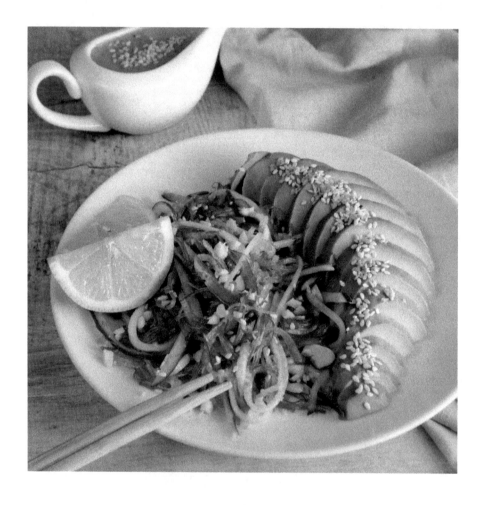

Broccoli and Cauliflower Mash

Preparation time: 2 minutes
Cooking time: 13 minutes
Servings: 3

Ingredients:
½ pound (227 g) broccoli florets
½ pound (227 g) cauliflower florets
Kosher salt and ground black pepper, to season
½ teaspoon garlic powder
1 teaspoon shallot powder
4 tablespoons whipped cream cheese
1½ tablespoons butter

Directions:
Microwave the broccoli and cauliflower for about 13 minutes until they have softened completely. Transfer to a food processor and add in the remaining ingredients.

Process the ingredients until everything is well combined.

Taste and adjust the seasoning. Bon appétit!

Nutrition:
calories 163, fat 12.8g, protein 4.7g, carbs 7.2g, net carbs 3.7g, fiber 3.5g

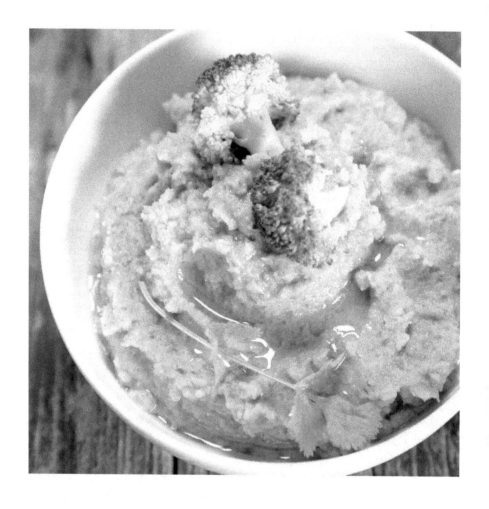

Sausage Frittata

Preparation time: 3 hours
Servings: 6

Ingredients:
6 oz sausages, chopped
6 eggs, beaten
¾ cup almond milk
teaspoon butter, melted
1 tablespoon dried parsley
½ teaspoon salt
1 oz Parmesan, grated

Directions:
Whisk the eggs and combine them with the chopped sausages.
Add almond milk and dried parsley.
Add the salt, grated cheese, and melted butter. Stir and pour into the slow cooker.
Close the lid and cook the meal for 3 hours on Low.
Enjoy!

Nutrition:
calories 249, fat 21.2g, fiber 0.7g, carbs 2.2g, protein 13.3g

Cheddar & Bacon Casserole

Preparation time: 10 minutes
Cooking time: 3 hours
Servings: 2

Ingredients:
5 ounces hash browns, shredded
bacon slices, cooked and chopped
ounces cheddar cheese, shredded
eggs, whisked
1 green onion, chopped
¼ cup milk
Cooking spray
A pinch of salt and black pepper

Directions:
Grease your slow cooker with cooking spray and add hash browns, bacon and cheese. In a bowl, mix eggs with green onion, milk, salt and pepper, whisk well and add to slow cooker. Cover, cook on High for 3 hours, divide between plates and serve. Enjoy!

Nutrition:
calories 281, fat 4g, fiber 6g, carbs 12g, protein 11g

Fish and Seafood

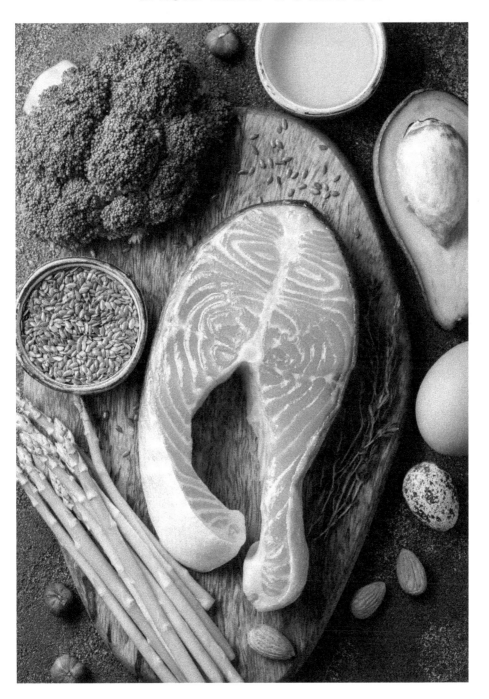

Coconut Shrimp Curry

Preparation Time: 10 minutes
Cooking Time: 2 hours 30 minutes
Serves: 4

Ingredients:
lb. shrimp
1/4 cup fresh cilantro, chopped
tsp. lemon garlic seasoning
1 Tbsp. curry paste
15 oz. water
30 oz. coconut milk

Directions:
Add coconut milk, cilantro, lemon garlic seasoning, curry paste, and water to a crock pot and stir well.
Cover and cook on high for 2 hours.
Add shrimp, cover and cook for 30 minutes longer.
Serve and enjoy.

Nutrition:
calories 200, fat 7.7g, carbohydrates 4.6g

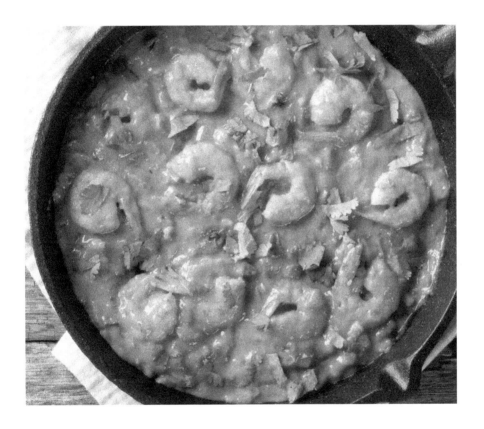

Slow Cooked Poached Salmon

Preparation time: 10 minutes
Cooking time: 6 hours
Servings: 4

Ingredients:
cup water
½ cup dry white wine
4 salmon fillets
1 sprig dill
1 yellow onion, sliced
1 lemon, sliced
½ teaspoon salt

Directions:
Add water and wine to the slow cooker and cook on HIGH for about 30-40 minutes.
Add rest of the ingredients and cook for 20-30 minutes more on HIGH or until salmon becomes opaque.
Serve hot or cold as per your liking.

Nutrition:
Calories 382, Fat 23 g, Carbs 4 g, Protein 35 g

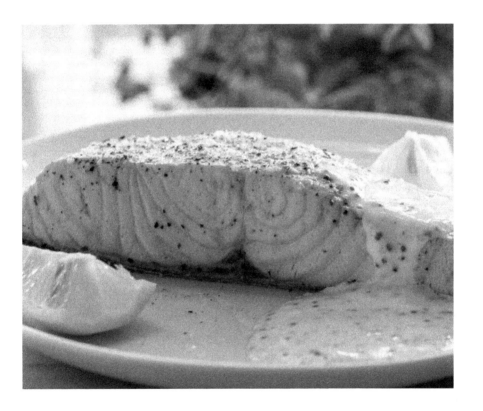

Creamy Kale Salad

Preparation Time: 15 minutes
Cooking Time: 0 minutes
Servings: 3

Ingredients:
1 bunch spinach
1 1/2 tablespoon lemon juice
1 cup sour cream
cup roasted macadamia
tablespoons sesame seeds oil
1/2 garlic clove, minced
1/2 teaspoon black pepper
1/4 teaspoon salt
tablespoons lime juice
1 bunch kale Toppings:
1 1/2 Avocado, diced
1/4 cup Pecans, chopped

Directions:
First of all, please confirm you've all the ingredients out there. Chop kale and wash kale then remove the ribs.
Now transfer kale to a large bowl.
One thing remains to be done. Add sour cream, lime juice, macadamia, sesame seeds oil, pepper, salt, garlic.
Finally, mix thoroughly. Top with your avocado and pecans. Serve& enjoy.

Nutrition:
calories 291, fat 5.1g, fiber 12.9g, carbohydrates 4.3 g, protein 11.8g

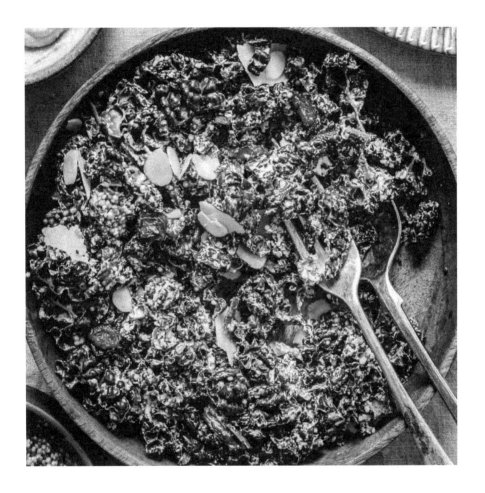

Trout Cakes

Preparation time: 10 minutes
Cooking time: 2 hours
Servings: 2

Ingredients:
7 oz. trout fillet, diced
1 tablespoon semolina
1 teaspoon dried oregano
¼ teaspoon ground black pepper
1 teaspoon corn flour
1 egg, beaten
1/3 cup water
1 teaspoon sesame oil

Directions:
In the bowl mix diced trout, semolina, dried oregano, ground black pepper, and corn flour.
Then add egg and carefully mix the mixture.
Heat the sesame oil well.
Then make the fish cakes and put them in the hot oil.
Roast them for 1 minute per side and transfer in the slow cooker.
Add water and cook the trout cakes for 2 hours on High.

Nutrition:
266 calories, 30g protein, 5.6g carbohydrates, 13.1g fat, 0.7g fiber, 155mg cholesterol, 99mg sodium, 519mg potassium

Slow Cooked Salmon Fillets

Preparation time: 10 minutes
Cooking time: 7 hours
Servings: 8

Ingredients:

4 salmon fillets, about 8 ounce each
tablespoons olive oil
¼ cup minced garlic
¼ cup onion, chopped
1 cup kidney beans, rinsed and drained
½ cup red bell pepper, diced
½ cup green bell pepper, diced
1 cup tomatoes, diced
1 cup tomato sauce
teaspoons chili powder
1 teaspoon ground cumin

Directions:

Sauté salmon fillets, olive oil, and onion for 8-10 minutes. Add the garlic, and stir until fragrant. Place cooked salmon fillets into the slow cooker with kidney beans, red bell pepper, green bell pepper, tomatoes, tomato sauce, chili powder, and cumin. Cook for 7 hours on low. Serve with baked potatoes or steamed rice.

Nutrition:

calories 293, fat 2.7 g, carbs 58.3 g, protein 14.9 g, dietary fiber 15.3 g, sugars 12.5 g

Shrimp Alfredo

Preparation Time: 15 minutes
Cooking Time: 30 minutes
Servings: 4

Ingredients:
1 pound of wild shrimp
3 tablespoons of organic grass-fed whey
1 1/2 cups of frozen asparagus
cup of heavy cream
1/2 cup of parmesan cheese
Sea salt
Black pepper
ground garlic cloves
1 small diced onion

Directions:
Peel and devein the shrimps, coat them well with salt and pepper. Let it cover in a bowl for 20 minutes.
Preheat a skillet. Put in butter, garlic, and onions.
When butter is melted, put in shrimp and stir fry till for 3 minutes.
Pour in heavy cream and stir well. Then, add ion cheese and stir till cheese melts.
Serve hot.

Nutrition:
calories 315, fat 11.9g, fiber 8.5g, carbohydrates 9.3 g, protein 11.1g

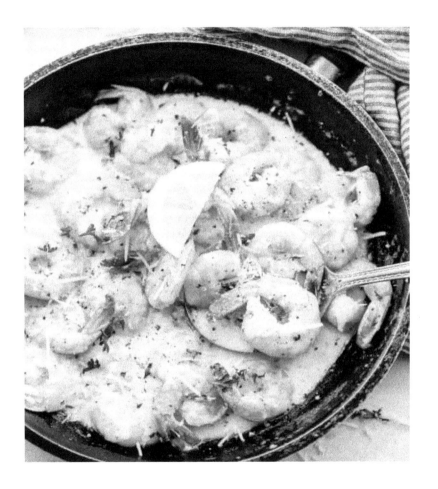

Haddock Chowder

Preparation time: 10 minutes
Cooking time: 6 hours
Servings: 5

Ingredients:
1-pound haddock, chopped
2 bacon slices, chopped, cooked
½ cup potatoes, chopped
1 teaspoon ground coriander
½ cup heavy cream
4 cups of water
1 teaspoon salt

Directions:
Put all ingredients in the slow cooker and close the lid.
Cook the chowder on Low for 6 hours.

Nutrition:
203 calories, 27.1g protein, 2.8g carbohydrates, 8.6g fat, 0.4g fiber,
97mg cholesterol, 737mg sodium, 506mg potassium

Blackened Salmon with Avocado Salsa

Preparation Time: 15 minutes
Cooking Time: 10 minutes
Servings: 4

Ingredients:

1 tbsp. extra virgin olive oil
4 filets of salmon (about 6 oz. each)
4 tsp. Cajun seasoning
2 med. avocados, diced
1 c. cucumber, diced
1/4 c. red onion, diced
1 tbsp. parsley, chopped
1 tbsp. lime juice
Sea salt & pepper, to taste

Directions:

The oil must be heated in a skillet. Rub the Cajun seasoning into the fillets, then lay them into the bottom of the skillet once it's hot enough. Cook until a dark crust forms, then flip and repeat. In a medium mixing bowl, combine all the ingredients for the salsa and set aside. Plate the fillets and top with 1/4 of the salsa yielded. Enjoy!

Nutrition:

calories 425, fat 15.8g, fiber 19.2g, carbohydrates 4.1 g, protein 11/8g

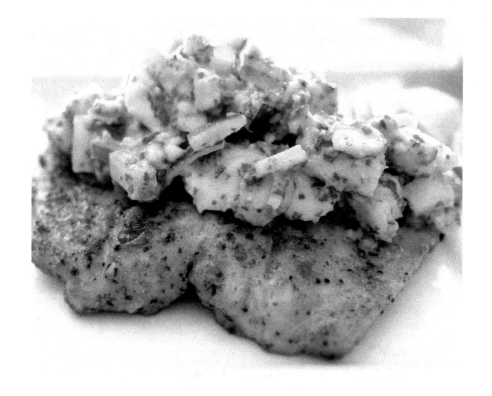

Braised Salmon

Preparation time: 10 minutes
Cooking time: 1 hours
Servings: 4

Ingredients:
1 cup of water
2-pound salmon fillet
1 teaspoon salt
1 teaspoon ground black pepper

Directions:
Put all ingredients in the slow cooker and close the lid.
Cook the salmon on High for 1 hour.

Nutrition:
301 calories, 44.1g protein, 0.3g carbohydrates, 14g fat, 0.1g fiber,
100mg Cholesterol, 683mg Sodium, 878mg Potassium

Sea bass Ragout

Preparation time: 15 minutes
Cooking time: 3.5 hours
Servings: 4

Ingredients:
7 oz. shiitake mushrooms
1 onion, diced
1 tablespoon coconut oil
1 teaspoon ground coriander
½ teaspoon salt
1 cup of water
12 oz. sea bass fillet, chopped

Directions:
Heat the coconut oil in the skillet.
Add onion and mushrooms and roast the vegetables for 5 minutes on medium heat.
Then transfer the vegetables in the slow cooker and add water.
Add fish fillet, salt, and ground coriander.
Cook the meal on High for 3.5 hours.

Nutrition:
241 calories, 20.4g protein, 9.4g carbohydrates, 14g fat, 2.3g fiber
0mg cholesterol, 413mg sodium, 99mg potassium

Alaska Cod with Butter Garlic Sauce

Preparation time: 10 minutes
Cooking time: 15 minutes
Servings: 6

Ingredients:
2 teaspoons olive oil
6 Alaska cod fillets
Salt and black pepper to taste
4 tablespoons salted butter
4 cloves garlic, minced
⅓ cup lemon juice
3 tablespoons white wine
2 tablespoons chopped chives

Directions:
Heat the oil in a skillet over medium heat and season the cod with salt and black pepper. Fry the fillets in the oil for 4 minutes on one side, flip and cook for 1 minute. Take out, plate, and set aside.
In another skillet over low heat, melt the butter and sauté the garlic for 3 minutes. Add the lemon juice, wine, and chives. Season with
salt, black pepper, and cook for 3 minutes until the wine slightly reduces. Put the fish in the skillet, spoon sauce over, cook for 30 seconds and turn the heat off.
Divide fish into 6 plates, top with sauce, and serve with buttered green beans.

Nutrition:
calories 265, fat 17.1g, protein 19.9g, carbs 2.5g, net carbs 2.4g, fiber 0.1g

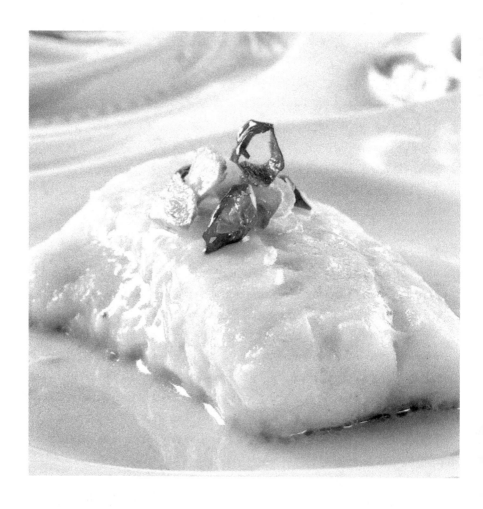

Coconut Mussels

Preparation Time: 10 minutes
Cooking Time: 10-15 minutes
Servings: 4

Ingredients:

2 tablespoons coconut oil
1/2 sweet onion, chopped
2 teaspoons minced garlic
1 teaspoon grated fresh ginger
1/2 teaspoon turmeric
1 cup of coconut milk
Juice of 1 lime
11/2 pounds fresh mussels, scrubbed and debearded
scallion, finely chopped
tablespoons chopped fresh cilantro
1 tablespoon chopped fresh thyme

Directions:

Sauté the aromatics. In a pot, warm the coconut oil. Add the onion, garlic, ginger, and turmeric and sauté until they've softened about 3 minutes. Add the liquid. Stir in the coconut milk and lime juice and bring the mixture to a boil. Steam the mussels.

Add the mussels to the skillet, cover, and steam until the shells are open, about 10 minutes. Take the skillet off the heat and throw out any unopened mussels. Add the herbs. Stir in the scallion, cilantro, and thyme. Serve. Divide the mussels and the sauce between four bowls and serve them immediately.

Nutrition:

calories 321, fat 11.1g, fiber 9g, carbohydrates 1.2 g, protein 1.4g

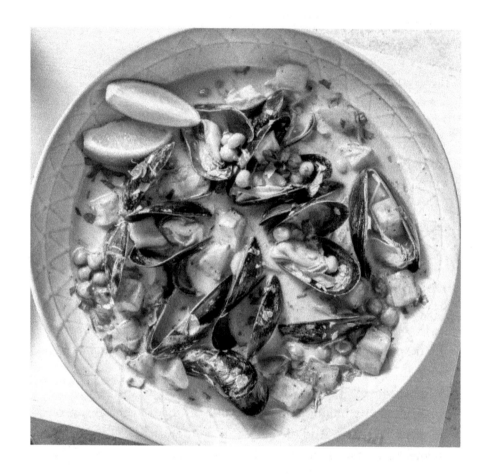

Tuna Cakes with Seeds

Preparation time: 10 minutes
Cooking time: 10 minutes
Servings: 4

Ingredients:
3 tablespoons sugar-free mayonnaise
1 tablespoon Sriracha sauce
1 teaspoon wheat-free soy sauce
1 teaspoon coconut flour
pound (454 g) fresh tuna, cut into ½-inch cubes
tablespoons white sesame seeds
tablespoon black sesame seeds
tablespoons avocado oil or other light-tasting oil, for the pan

Directions:
In a mixing bowl, whisk together the mayonnaise, Sriracha, soy sauce, and flour until smooth. Add the tuna and stir to combine.
Combine the white and black sesame seeds and spread on a small plate.
Using your hands, form the tuna mixture into 12 small cakes about 2 inches in diameter. Gently dip both sides of the cakes in the sesame seeds to lightly coat them.
Heat the oil in a medium-sized nonstick sauté pan over medium heat. Cook the cakes in batches, 1 to 2 minutes per side, until golden brown. Serve warm.

Nutrition:
calories 300, fat 18.9g, protein 26.9g, carbs 2.0g, net carbs 1.0g, fiber 1.0g

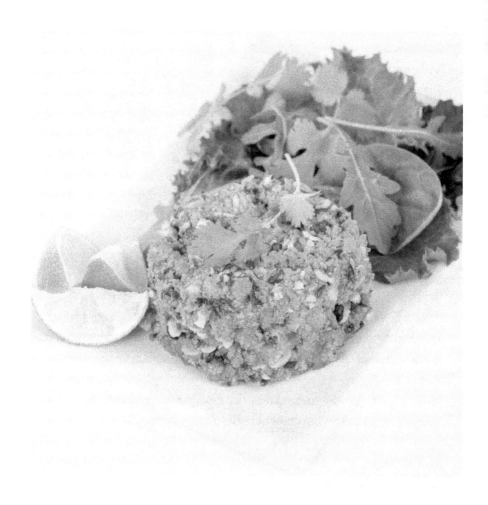

Chimichurri Grilled Shrimp

Preparation time: 10 minutes
Cooking time: 35 minutes
Servings: 4

Ingredients:
pound (454 g)shrimp, peeled and deveined
tablespoons olive oil
Juice of 1 lime
Chimichurri:
½ teaspoon salt
¼ cup olive oil
2 garlic cloves
¼ cup red onions, chopped
¼ cup red wine vinegar
½ teaspoon pepper
2 cups parsley
¼ teaspoon red pepper flakes

Directions:
Process the chimichurri ingredients in a blender until smooth; set aside.
Combine shrimp, olive oil, and lime juice, in a bowl, and let marinate in the
fridge for 30 minutes. Preheat your grill to medium. Add shrimp and cook
about 2 minutes per side. Serve shrimp drizzled with the chimichurri sauce.

Nutrition:
calories 284, fat 20.4g, protein 15.8g, carbs 4.8g, net carbs 3.6g, fiber 1.2g

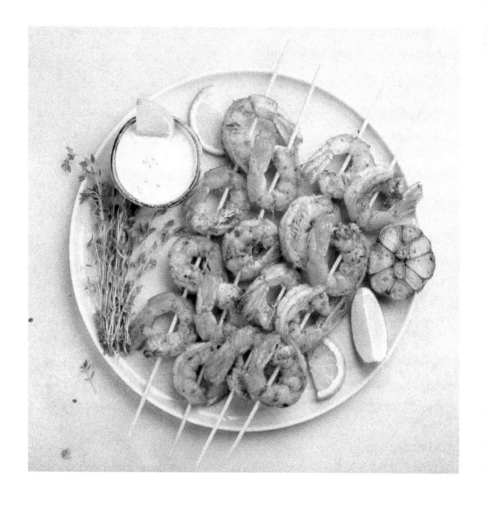

Parmesan-Garlic Salmon with Asparagus

Preparation Time: 10 minutes
Cooking Time: 15 minutes
Servings: 2

Ingredients:
(6-ounce) salmon fillets, skin on
Pink Himalayan salt
Freshly ground black pepper
1-pound fresh asparagus ends snapped off
tablespoons butter
2 garlic cloves, minced
1/4 cup grated Parmesan cheese

Directions:
Oven: 400°F. Pat the salmon dry and season both sides with pink Himalayan salt and pepper. Put the salmon, and arrange the asparagus around the salmon. Melt the butter. Add the minced garlic and stir until the garlic just begins to brown about 3 minutes. Drizzle the garlic-butter sauce over the salmon and asparagus, and top both with the Parmesan cheese. Bake until the salmon is cooked and the asparagus is crisp-tender, about 12 minutes. You can switch the oven to broil at the end of cooking time to char the asparagus. Serve hot.

Nutrition:
calories 476, fat 14.1g, fiber 10.5g, carbohydrates 3.1 g, protein 19.9g

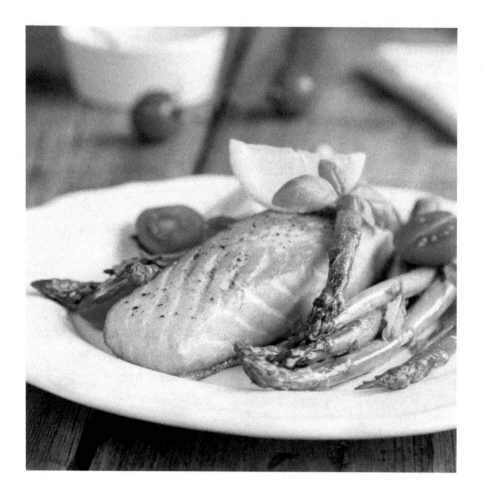

Creamy Herbed Salmon

Preparation time: 10 minutes
Cooking time: 10 minutes
Servings: 2

Ingredients:
2 salmon fillets
¾ teaspoon dried tarragon
2 tablespoons olive oil
¾ teaspoon dried dill
Sauce:
2 tablespoons butter
½ teaspoon dill
½ teaspoon tarragon
¼ cup heavy cream
Salt and black pepper to taste

Directions:
Season the salmon with dill and tarragon. Warm the olive oil in a pan over medium heat. Add salmon and cook for about 4 minutes on both sides. Set aside.
To make the sauce: melt the butter and add the dill and tarragon. Cook for 30 seconds to infuse the flavors. Whisk in the heavy cream, season with salt and black pepper, and cook for 2-3 minutes. Serve the salmon topped with the sauce.

Nutrition:
calories 467, fat 40.1g, protein 22.1g, carbs 1.9g, net carbs 1.6g, fiber 0.3g

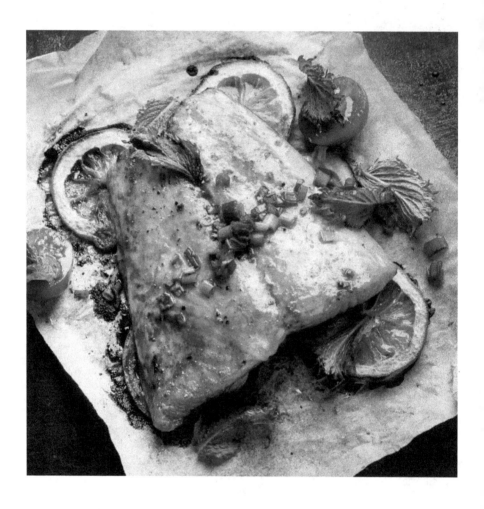

Fennel and Trout Parcels

Preparation time: 10 minutes
Cooking time: 15 minutes
Servings: 4

Ingredients:
½ pound (227 g) deboned trout, butterflied
Salt and black pepper to season
tablespoons olive oil plus extra for tossing
sprigs rosemary
4 sprigs thyme
4 butter cubes
1 cup thinly sliced fennel
1 medium red onion, sliced
8 lemon slices
3 teaspoons capers to garnish

Directions:
Preheat the oven to 400°F (205°C). Cut out parchment paper wide enough for each trout. In a bowl, toss the fennel and onion with a little bit of olive oil and share into the middle parts of the papers.
Place the fish on each veggie mound, top with a drizzle of olive oil each, a pinch of salt and black pepper, a sprig of rosemary and thyme, and 1 cube of butter. Also, lay the lemon slices on the fish. Wrap and close the fish packets securely, and place them on a baking sheet.
Bake in the oven for 15 minutes, and remove once ready. Plate them and garnish the fish with capers and serve with a squash mash.

Nutrition:
calories 235, fat 9.1g, protein 17.1g, carbs 3.7g, net carbs 2.7g, fiber 1.0g

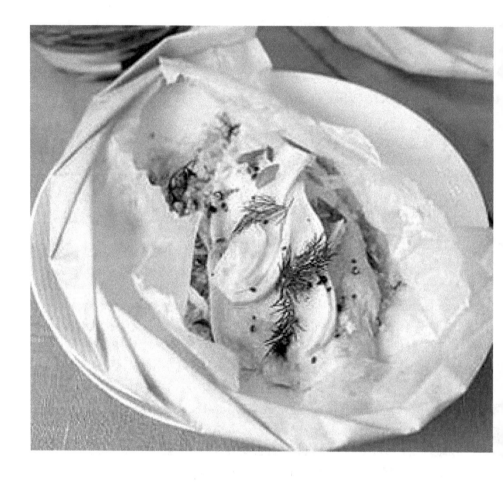

Scallops with Creamy Bacon Sauce

Preparation Time: 5 minutes
Cooking Time: 20 minutes
Servings: 2

Ingredients:
4 bacon slices
1 cup heavy (whipping) cream
1 tablespoon butter
1/4 cup grated Parmesan cheese
Pink Himalayan salt
Freshly ground black pepper
1 tablespoon ghee
8 large sea scallops, rinsed and patted dry

Directions:
Cook the bacon. Lower the heat to medium. Add the butter, cream, and Parmesan cheese to the bacon grease and season with a pinch of pink Himalayan salt and pepper. Lower the heat down, then stir constantly until the sauce thickens and is reduced by 50 percent, about 10 minutes. In another skillet, heat the ghee until sizzling. Season the scallops with pink Himalayan salt and pepper, and add them to the skillet—Cook for just 1 minute per side. Do not crowd the scallops; if your pan isn't large enough, cook them in two batches. You want the scallops golden on each side. Transfer the scallops to a paper towel-lined plate. Divide the cream sauce between two plates, crumble the bacon on top of the cream sauce, and top with four scallops. Serve immediately.

Nutrition:
alories 311, fat 14.1g, fiber 10.3g, carbohydrates 1.2 g, protein 17.7g

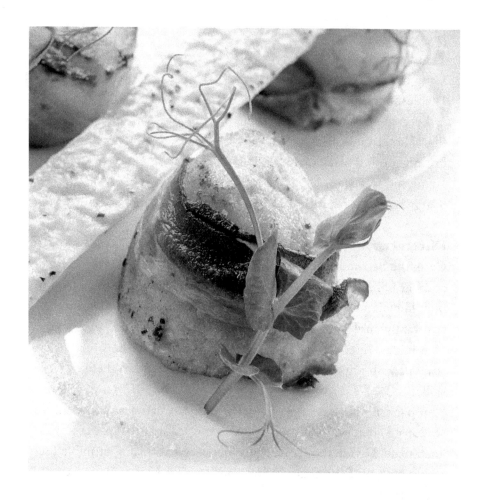

Almond Breaded Hoki

Preparation time: 15 minutes
Cooking time: 25 minutes
Servings: 4

Ingredients:
1 cup flaked smoked hoki, bones removed
1 cup cubed hoki fillets, cubed
4 eggs
1 cup water
3 tablespoons almond flour
onion, sliced
cups sour cream
1 tablespoon chopped parsley
1 cup pork rinds, crushed
cup grated Cheddar cheese
Salt and black pepper to taste
tablespoons butter

Directions:

Preheat the oven to 360°F (182°C) and lightly grease a baking dish with cooking spray. Then, boil the eggs in water in a pot over medium heat to be well done for 10 minutes, run the eggs under cold water and peel the shells. After, place on a cutting board and chop them.

Melt the butter in a saucepan over medium heat and sauté the onion for 4 minutes. Turn the heat off and stir in the almond flour to form a roux. Turn the heat back on and cook the roux to be golden brown and stir in the cream until the mixture is smooth. Season with salt and black pepper, and stir in the parsley.

Spread the smoked and cubed fish in the baking dish, sprinkle the eggs on top, and spoon the sauce over. In a bowl, mix the pork rinds with the Cheddar cheese, and sprinkle it over the sauce.

Bake the casserole in the oven for 20 minutes until the top is golden and the sauce and cheese are bubbly. Remove the bake after and serve with a steamed green vegetable mix.

Nutrition:

calories 384, fat 27.1g, protein 28.4g, carbs 3.9g, net carbs 3.6g, fiber 0.3g

Tomato and Olive Tilapia Flillets

Preparation time: 10 minutes
Cooking time: 25 minutes
Servings: 4

Ingredients:

4 tilapia fillets
2 garlic cloves, minced
2 teaspoons oregano
14 ounces (397 g) diced tomatoes
tablespoon olive oil
½ red onion, chopped
tablespoons parsley
¼ cup kalamata olives

Directions:

Heat olive oil in a skillet over medium heat and cook the onion for 3 minutes.
Add garlic and oregano and cook for 30 seconds. Stir in tomatoes and bring the
mixture to a boil. Reduce the heat and simmer for 5 minutes. Add olives and
tilapia, and cook for about 8 minutes. Serve the tilapia with tomato sauce.

Nutrition:

calories 283, fat 15.1g, protein 22.9g, carbs 7.9g, net carbs 5.9g, fiber 2.0g

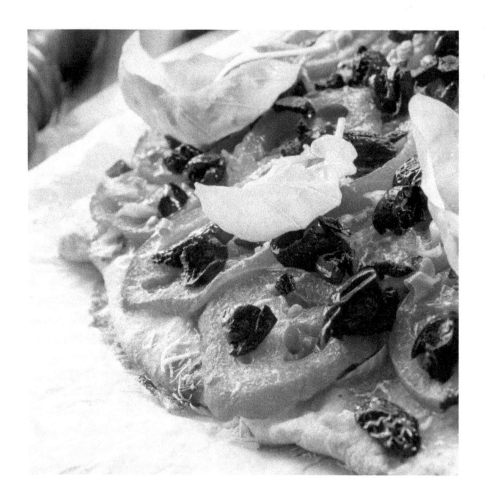

Curried Fish with Super Greens

Preparation Time: 10 minutes
Cooking Time: 20 minutes
Servings: 4

Ingredients:
2 tablespoons coconut oil
2 teaspoons garlic, minced
11/2 tablespoons grated fresh ginger
1/2 teaspoon ground cumin
tablespoon curry powder
cups of coconut milk
16 ounces (454 g) firm white fish, cut into 1-inch chunks
cup kale, shredded
tablespoons cilantro, chopped

Directions:
Melt the coconut oil in a heated pan. Add the garlic and ginger and
sauté for about 2 minutes until tender. Fold in the cumin and curry
powder, then cook for 1 to 2 minutes until fragrant. Put in the coconut
milk and boil. Boil then simmer until the flavors mellow, about 5
minutes. Add the fish chunks and simmer for 10 minutes until the fish
flakes easily with a fork, stirring once. Scatter the shredded kale and
chopped cilantro over the fish, then cook for 2 minutes more until
softened.

Nutrition:
calories 376, fat 19.9g, fiber 15.8g, carbohydrates 6.7 g, protein 14.8 g

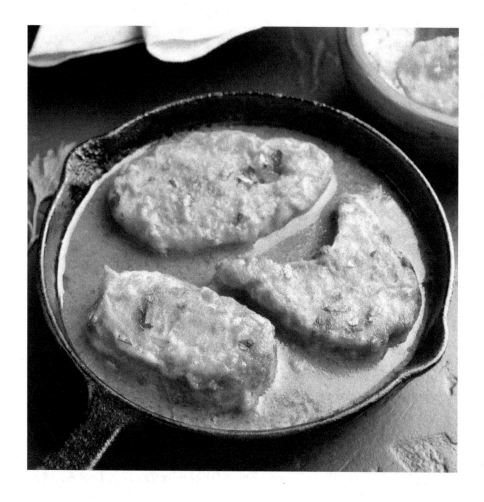

Soup

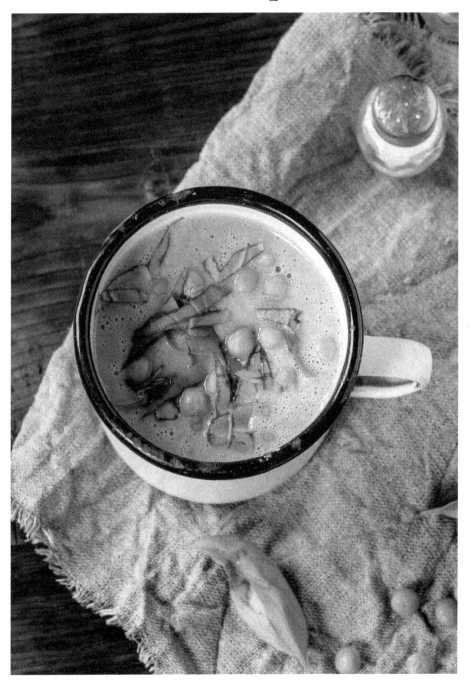

Celery Soup with Ham

Preparation time: 10 minutes
Cooking time: 5 hours
Servings: 8

Ingredients:

8 oz. ham, chopped
8 cups chicken stock
teaspoon white pepper
½ teaspoon cayenne pepper
cups celery stalk, chopped
½ cup corn kernels

Directions:

Put all ingredients in the slow cooker and gently stir.
Close the lid and cook the soup on High for 5 hours.
When the soup is cooked, cool it to the room temperature and ladle
into the bowls.

Nutrition:

69 calories, 5.9g protein, 4.6g carbohydrates, 3.2g fat, 1.1g fiber,
16mg cholesterol, 1155mg sodium, 193mg potassium

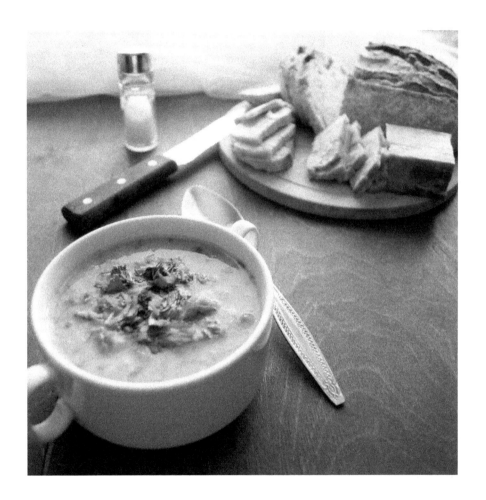

Sauerkraut and Organic Sausage Soup

Preparation time: 15 minutes
Cooking time: 6 hours
Servings: 6

Ingredients:
1 tablespoon extra-virgin olive oil
6 cups beef broth
pound (454 g) organic sausage, cooked and sliced
cups sauerkraut
2 celery stalks, chopped
sweet onion, chopped
teaspoons minced garlic
2 tablespoons butter
tablespoon hot mustard
½ teaspoon caraway seeds
½ cup sour cream
tablespoons chopped fresh parsley, for garnish

Directions:
Lightly grease the insert of the slow cooker with the olive oil.
Place the broth, sausage, sauerkraut, celery, onion, garlic, butter, mustard, and
caraway seeds in the insert.
Cover and cook on low for 6 hours.
Stir in the sour cream.
Serve topped with the parsley.

Nutrition:
calories 333, fat 27.9g, protein 15.2g, carbs 5.9g, net carbs 2.0g, fiber 3.9g

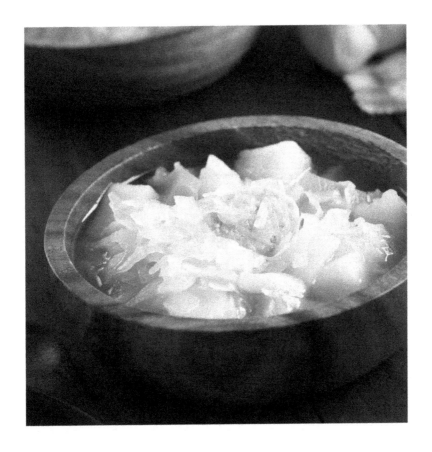

Cheesy Coconut Carrot Soup

Preparation time: 15 minutes
Cooking time: 6 hours
Servings: 6

Ingredients:
1 tablespoon butter
5 cups chicken broth
cup coconut milk
celery stalks, chopped
1 carrot, chopped
½ sweet onion, chopped
Pinch cayenne pepper
8 ounces (227 g) cream cheese, cubed
2 cups shredded Cheddar cheese
Salt, for seasoning
Freshly ground black pepper, for seasoning
1 tablespoon chopped fresh thyme, for garnish

Directiions:
Lightly grease the insert of the slow cooker with the butter.
Place the broth, coconut milk, celery, carrot, onion, and cayenne pepper in the insert.
Cover and cook on low for 6 hours.
Stir in the cream cheese and Cheddar, then season with salt and pepper.
Serve topped with the thyme.

Nutrition:
calories 405, fat 36.0g, protein 14.9g, carbs 6.9g, net carbs 5.9g, fiber 1.0g

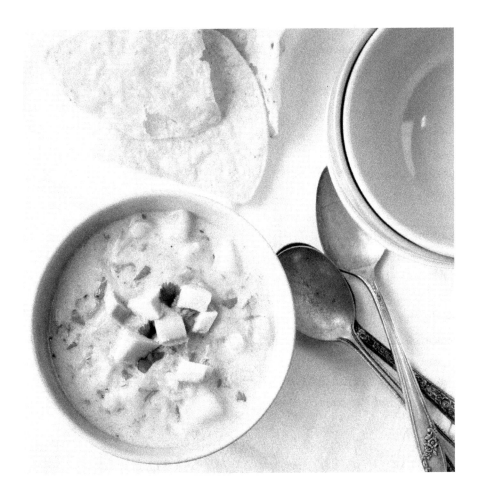

Chicken Garlic Soup

Preparation time: 10 minutes
Cooking time: 15 minutes
Servings: 6

Ingredients:

2 boneless, skinless chicken breasts
4 cups chicken broth
½ cup whipped cream cheese
3 cloves garlic, chopped
1 teaspoon thyme
1 teaspoon salt
¼ teaspoon black pepper
1 tablespoon butter

Directions:

Preheat a stockpot over medium heat with the butter.
Add the chicken and brown until completely cooked through. Remove from heat.
Shred the chicken and add it back to the stockpot along with the remaining ingredients minus the cream cheese.
Bring to a simmer.
Add in the cream cheese and whisk until there are no more clumps.
Simmer for 10 minutes and serve.

Nutrition:

calories 130, fat 6.1g, protein 15.9g, carbs 2.1g, net carbs 2.1g, fiber 0g

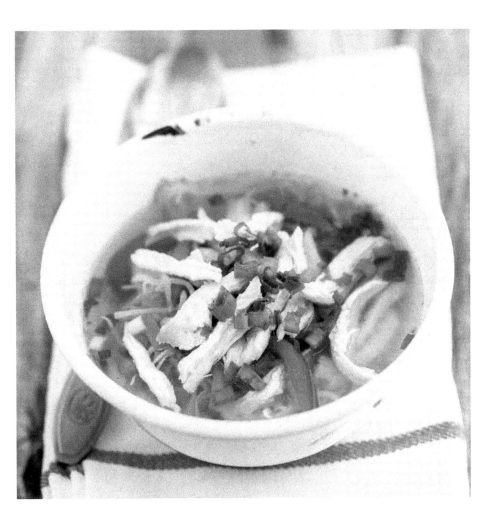

Beef Stock

Preparation time: 5 minutes
Cooking time: 8 hours
Servings: 2

Ingredients:
2 pounds beef bones
1 carrot, halved ½ yellow onion
1 tablespoon canola oil
1 celery stalk, halved
1 teaspoon black peppercorns
½ teaspoon sea salt
1 gallon water

Directions:
Preheat the oven to 375°F.
On a rimmed baking sheet, coat the beef bones, carrot, and onion in the oil. Spread them out in an even layer. Transfer the baking sheet to the oven. Roast for 35 to 45 minutes, turning the bones occasionally. (Do not let them burn.) Remove from the oven. Transfer the roasted bones, carrot, and onion to the slow cooker. Add the celery, peppercorns, salt, and water. Stir, then cover and cook on low for 8 to 10 hours.
Turn off the slow cooker. Strain the stock through a fine-mesh sieve. Discard the vegetables. Store the stock in a covered container in the refrigerator for up to 4 days or in the freezer for up to 3 months.

Nutrition:
calories 12, total fat 0g, saturated fat 0g, carbohydrates 1g, sodium 73mg, fiber: 0g, protein 2g

Italian Pork Sausage and Zoodle Soup

Preparation time: 15 minutes
Cooking time: 25 minutes
Servings: 8

Ingredients:
1 tablespoon olive oil
4 cloves garlic, minced
1 pound (454 g) pork sausage (no sugar added)
½ tablespoon Italian seasoning
3 cups regular beef broth
3 cups beef bone broth
2 medium zucchini (6 ounces / 170 g each), spiralized

Directions:
In a large soup pot, heat the oil over medium heat. Add the garlic and cook for about 1 minute, until fragrant.
Add the sausage, increase the heat to medium-high, and cook for about 10 minutes, stirring occasionally and breaking apart into small pieces, until browned.
Add the seasoning, regular broth, and bone broth, and simmer for 10 minutes.
Add the zucchini. Bring to a simmer again, then simmer for about 2 minutes, until the zucchini is soft. (Don't overcook or the zoodles will be mushy.)

Nutrition:
calories 215, fat 16.8g, protein 12.2g, carbs 2.1, net carbs 2.1g, fiber 0g

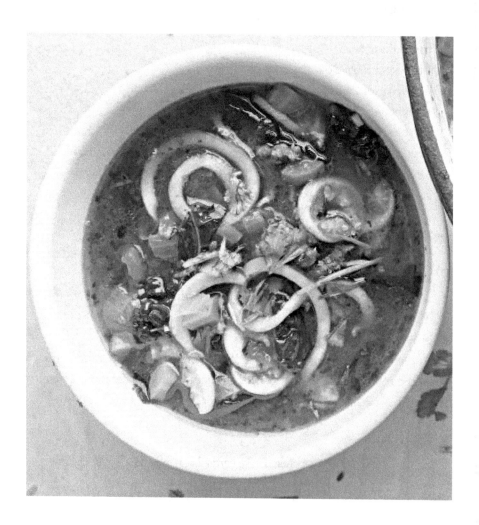

Light Zucchini Soup

Preparation time: 15 minutes
Cooking time: 30 minutes
Servings: 4

Ingredients:
1 large zucchini
1 white onion, diced
4 cups beef broth
1 teaspoon dried thyme
½ teaspoon dried rosemary

Directions:
Pour the beef broth in the slow cooker.
Add onion, dried thyme, and dried rosemary.
After this, make the spirals from the zucchini with the help of the paralyzer and transfer them in the slow cooker.
Close the lid and cook the soul on High for 30 minutes.

Nutrition:
64 calories, 6.2g protein, 6.5g carbohydrates, 1.6g fat, 1.6g fiber, 0mg cholesterol, 773mg sodium, 462mg potassium

Snacks and Appetizer

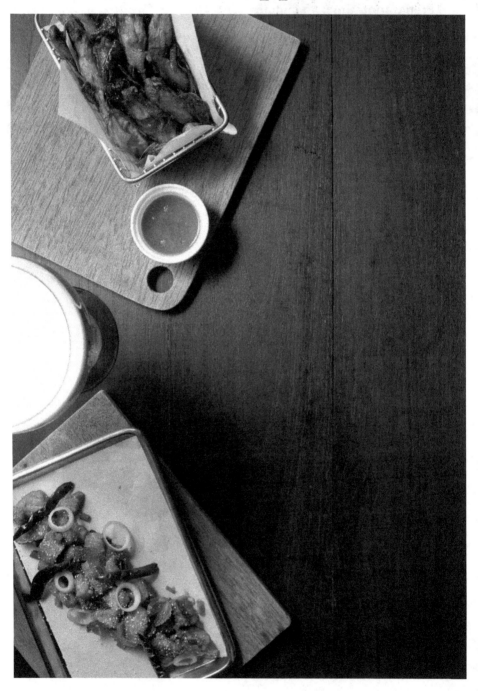

Crab Dip

Preparation time: 10 minutes
Cooking time: 1 hour
Servings: 2

Ingredients:
ounces crabmeat
tablespoon lime zest, grated
½ tablespoon lime juice
tablespoons mayonnaise
2 green onions, chopped
2 ounces cream cheese, cubed
Cooking spray

Directions:
Grease your slow cooker with the cooking spray, and mix the crabmeat with the lime zest, juice and the other ingredients inside.
Put the lid on, cook on Low for 1 hour, divide into bowls and serve as a party dip.

Nutrition:
calories 100, fat 3g, fiber 2g, carbs 9g, protein 4g

Bakery Mini Almond Muffins

Preparation time: 15 minutes
Cooking time: 20 minutes
Servings: 9

Ingredients:

3 eggs
tablespoons coconut oil
ounces (85 g) double cream
1 cup almond meal
½ cup flax seed meal
½ teaspoon monk fruit powder
½ teaspoon baking soda
½ teaspoon baking powder
A pinch of salt
½ teaspoon ground cloves
1 teaspoon ground cinnamon
1 teaspoon vanilla essence

Directions:

In a mixing bowl, whisk the eggs with the coconut milk and double cream.
In another bowl, mix the remaining ingredients. Now, add the wet mixture to
the dry mixture. Mix again to combine well.
Spoon the batter into small silicone molds. Bake in the preheated oven at 360°F
(182°C) for 13 to 17 minutes. Bon appétit!

Nutrition:

calories 86, fat 6.5g, protein 4.2g, carbs 3.2g, net carbs 3.2g, fiber 0g

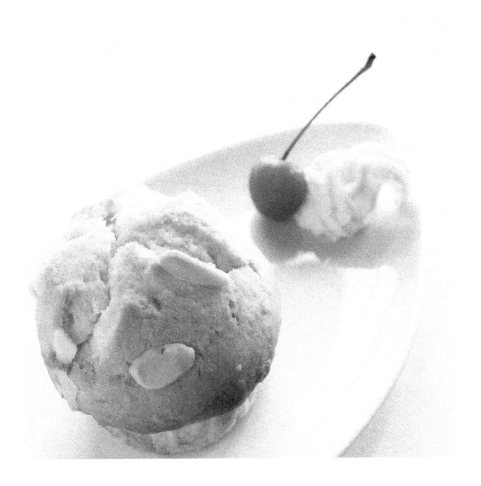

Corn Dip

Preparation time: 10 minutes
Cooking time: 3 hours
Servings: 12

Ingredients:
9 cups corn, rice and wheat cereal
cup cheerios
cups pretzels
1 cup peanuts
6 tablespoons hot, melted butter
1 tablespoon salt
¼ cup Worcestershire sauce
1 teaspoon garlic powder

Directions:
In your slow cooker, mix cereal with cheerios, pretzels, peanuts, butter, salt, Worcestershire sauce and garlic powder, toss well, cover and cook on Low for 3 hours.
Divide into bowls and serve as a snack.

Nutrition:
calories 182, fat 4g, fiber 5g, carbs 8g, protein 8g

Chicken Wrapped Provolone and Prosciutto

Preparation time: 10 minutes
Cooking time: 10 minutes
Servings: 8

Ingredients:
¼ teaspoon garlic powder
8 ounces (227 g) provolone cheese
8 raw chicken tenders
Black pepper to taste
8 prosciutto slices

Directions:
Pound the chicken until half an inch thick. Season with salt, pepper, and garlic powder. Cut the provolone cheese into 8 strips. Place a slice of prosciutto on a flat surface. Place one chicken tender on top. Top with a provolone strip. Roll the chicken, and secure with previously soaked skewers.Preheat the grill. Grill the wraps for about 3 minutes per side.

Nutrition:
calories 175, fat 10.1g, protein 16.9g, carbs 0g, net carbs 0.7g, fiber 0g

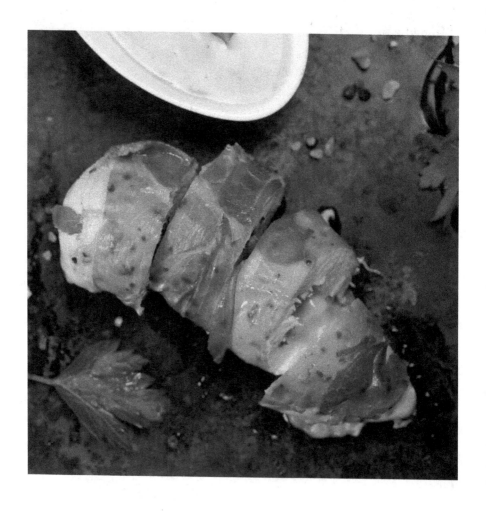

Mexican Dip

Preparation time: 10 minutes
Cooking time: 1 hour and 30 minutes
Servings: 10

Ingredients:
24 ounces cream cheese, cubed
cups rotisserie chicken breast, shredded
ounces canned green chilies, chopped
1 and ½ cups Monterey jack cheese, shredded
1 and ½ cups salsa Verde
1 tablespoon green onions, chopped

Directions:
In your slow cooker, mix cream cheese with chicken, chilies, cheese, salsa Verde and green onions, stir, cover and cook on Low for 1 hour and 30 minutes. Divide into bowls and serve.

Nutrition:
calories 222, fat 4g, fiber 5g, carbs 15g, protein 4g

Cheese Biscuits

Preparation time: 15 minutes
Cooking time: 20 minutes
Servings: 10

Ingredients:
1 cup coconut flour
½ cup flaxseed meal
1½ cups almond meal
½ teaspoon baking soda
1 teaspoon baking powder
½ teaspoon salt
teaspoon paprika
eggs
1 stick butter
1 cup Romano cheese, grated
1½ cups Colby cheese, grated

Directions:
Mix the flour with the baking soda, baking powder, salt, and paprika. In a separate bowl, beat the eggs and butter. Stir the wet mixture into the flour mixture. Fold in the grated cheese. Mix again until everything is well incorporated.
Roll the batter into 16 balls and place them on a lightly greased cookie sheet. Flatten them slightly with the palms of your hands.
Bake at 350°F (180°C) for about 17 minutes. Bon appétit!

Nutrition:
calories 380, fat 33.6g, protein 14.0g, carbs 6.6g, net carbs 1.6g, fiber 5.0g

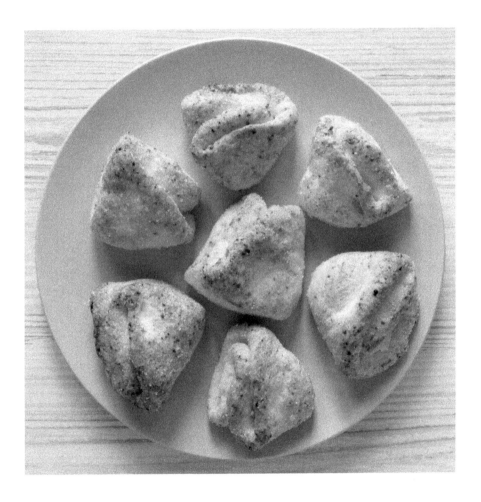

Party Snack Mix

Preparation time: 15 minutes
Cooking time: 2 hours
Servings: 8

Ingredients:
4 cups rice Chex cereal
cup corn Chex cereal
cups small pretzels
cup shelled peanuts
tablespoons unsalted butter, melted, or extra-virgin olive oil
1 teaspoon smoked paprika
1 teaspoon garlic powder
1 teaspoon onion powder
1 teaspoon minced fresh rosemary (optional)
1 tablespoon vegetarian Worcestershire sauce

Directions:
Place the rice cereal, corn cereal, pretzels, and peanuts in a 3-quart slow cooker. Stir to combine. In a small measuring cup, whisk together the butter, paprika, garlic powder, onion powder, rosemary (if using), and Worcestershire sauce. Pour this mixture into the slow cooker on top of the cereal mixture and stir gently to thoroughly coat. Cook on low, uncovered, for 2 hours. Stir several times to ensure that the mixture cooks evenly and does not stick to the slow cooker. The mix is done when the cereal is glazed. Remove the mix from the slow cooker, spread it onto a parchment paper– lined baking sheet, and let cool for 2 hours before serving or storing.

Nutrition:
calories 121, fat 6g, saturated fat 2g, cholesterol 4mg, carbohydrates 14g, fiber 1g, protein 3g, sodium 164mg

Dessert

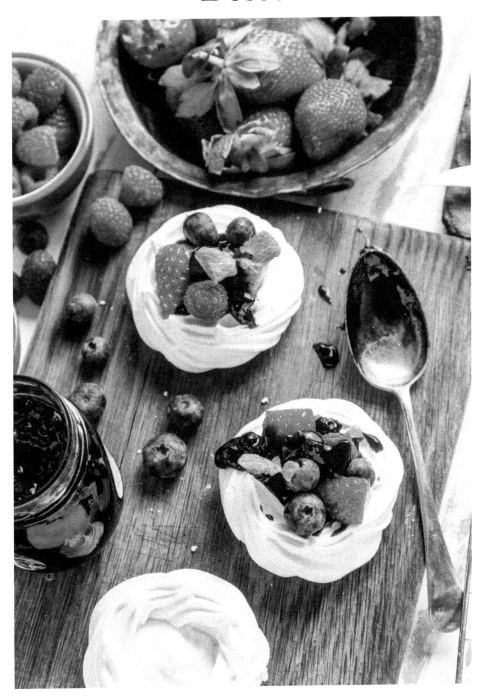

Almonds, Walnuts and Mango Bowls

Preparation time: 10 minutes
Cooking time: 2 hours
Servings: 2

Ingredients:
cup walnuts, chopped
tablespoons almonds, chopped
1 cup mango, peeled and roughly cubed
1 cup heavy cream
½ teaspoon vanilla extract
1 teaspoon almond extract
1 tablespoon brown sugar

Directions:
In your slow cooker, mix the nuts with the mango, cream and the other ingredients, toss, put the lid on and cook on High for 2 hours.
Divide the mix into bowls and serve.

Nutrition:
calories 220, fat 4g, fiber 2g, carbs 4g, protein 6g

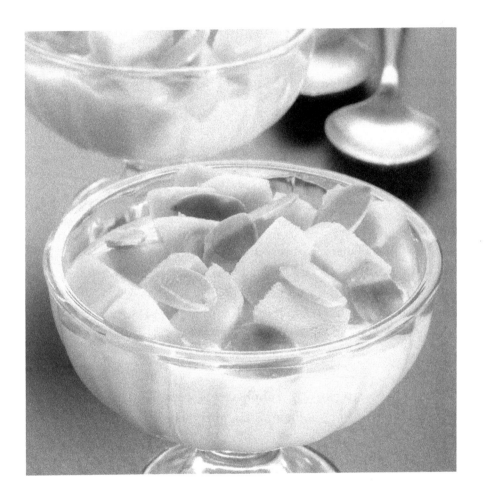

Dump Cake

Preparation time: 15 minutes
Cooking time: 5 hours
Servings: 8

Ingredients:
1 cupcake mix
teaspoon vanilla extract
½ teaspoon ground nutmeg
1 tablespoon butter, melted
eggs, beaten
1 teaspoon lemon zest, grated
½ cup heavy cream
4 pecans, chopped

Directions:
In the bowl mix all ingredients except pecans.
The line the slow cooker with baking paper and pour the dough inside.
Flatten the batter and top with pecans.
Close the lid and cook the dump cake for 5 hours on Low.
Cook the cooked cake well before serving.

Nutrition:
245 calories, 3.8g protein, 27g carbohydrates, 13.9g fat, 1.1g fiber, 55mg cholesterol, 246mg sodium, 90mg potassium

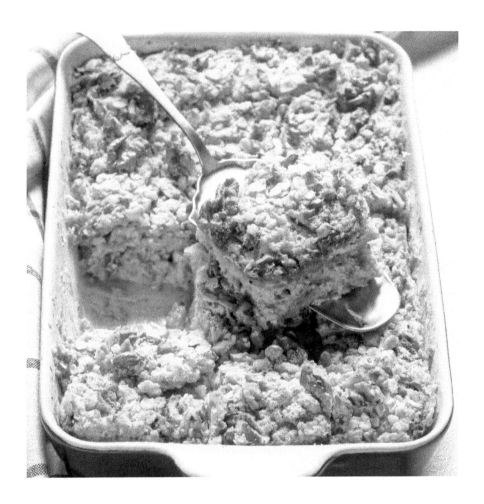

Easy Monkey Rolls

Preparation time: 15 minutes
Cooking time: 3 hours
Servings: 8

Ingredients:
tablespoon liquid honey
tablespoon sugar
eggs, beaten
1-pound cinnamon rolls, dough
tablespoons butter, melted

Directions:
Cut the cinnamon roll dough on 8 servings.
Then line the bottom of the slow cooker with baking paper and put the rolls inside.
In the bowl mix sugar, egg, liquid honey, and butter. Whisk the mixture.
Pour the egg mixture over the cinnamon roll dough and flatten well.
Close the lid and cook the meal on High for 3 hours.

Nutrition:
266 calories, 4.9g protein, 32.6g carbohydrates, 13.3g fat, 1.4g fiber, 86mg cholesterol, 253mg sodium, 80mg potassium

Apricot Spoon Cake

Preparation time: 15 minutes
Cooking time: 2.5 hours
Servings: 10

Ingredients:
2 cups cake mix
1 cup milk
cup apricots, canned, pitted, chopped, with juice
eggs, beaten
1 tablespoon sunflower oil

Directions:
Mix milk with cake mix and egg. Then sunflower oil and blend the mixture until smooth. Then place the baking paper in the slow cooker. Pour the cake mix batter in the slow cooker, flatten it gently, and close the lid. Cook the cake on High for 2.5 hours.
Then transfer the cooked cake in the plate and top with apricots and apricot juice.
Leave the cake until it is warm and cut into servings.

Nutrition:
268 calories, 4.5g protein, 43.8g carbohydrates, 8.6g fat, 0.8g fiber, 35mg cholesterol, 372mg sodium, 127mg potassium

Berry Marmalade

Preparation time: 10 minutes
Cooking time: 3 hours
Servings: 12

Ingredients:
1 pound cranberries
pound strawberries
½ pound blueberries
3.5ounces black currant
pounds sugar
Zest of 1 lemon 2 tablespoon water

Directions:
In your slow cooker, mix strawberries with cranberries, blueberries, currants, lemon zest, sugar and water, cover, cook on High for 3 hours, divide into jars and serve cold.

Nutrition:
calories 100, fat 4g, fiber 3g, carbs 12g, protein 3g

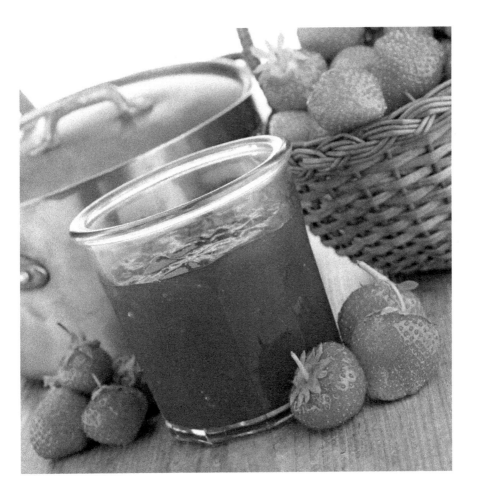

Rum Brownies

Preparation time: 15 minutes
Cooking time: 22 minutes
Serviings: 8

Ingredients:
⅔ cup almond flour
½ cup coconut flour
1 teaspoon baking powder
cup xylitol
½ cup cocoa powder, unsweetened
eggs
6 ounces (170 g) butter, melted
3 ounces (85 g) baking chocolate, unsweetened and melted
2 tablespoons rum
A pinch of salt
A pinch of freshly grated nutmeg
¼ teaspoon ground cinnamon

Directions:
In a mixing bowl, thoroughly combine dry ingredients. In a separate bowl, mix all the wet ingredients until well combined.
Stir dry mixture into wet ingredients. Evenly spread the batter into a parchment-lined baking dish.
Bake in the preheated oven at 360°F (182°C) for 20 to 22 minutes, until your brownies are set. Cut into squares and serve.

Nutrition:
calories 321, fat 30.1g, protein 5.7g, carbs 6.2g, net carbs 2.6g, fiber 3.6g

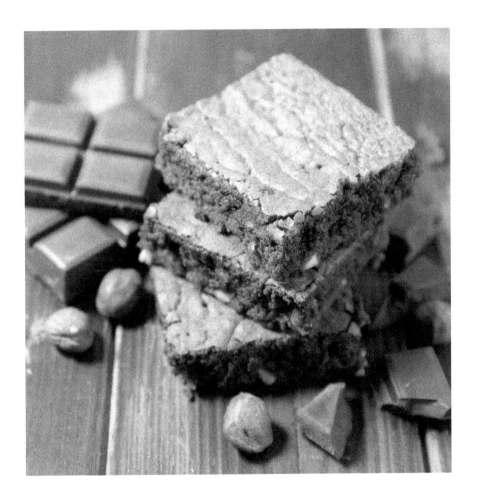

Peanut and Chocolate Balls

Preparation time: 15 minutes
Cooking time: 0 minutes
Servings: 6

Ingredients:

½ cup coconut oil
½ cup peanut butter, no sugar added
¼ cup cocoa powder, unsweetened
¼ cup Xylitol
4 tablespoons roasted peanuts, ground

Directions:

Microwave the coconut oil until melted; add in the peanut butter and stir until well combined.

Add the cocoa powder and Xylitol to the batter. Transfer to your freezer for about 1 hour.

Shape the batter into bite-sized balls and roll them over the ground peanuts. Bon appétit!

Nutrition:

calories 330, fat 32.5g, protein 6.8g, carbs 7.5g, net carbs 4.9g, fiber 2.6g

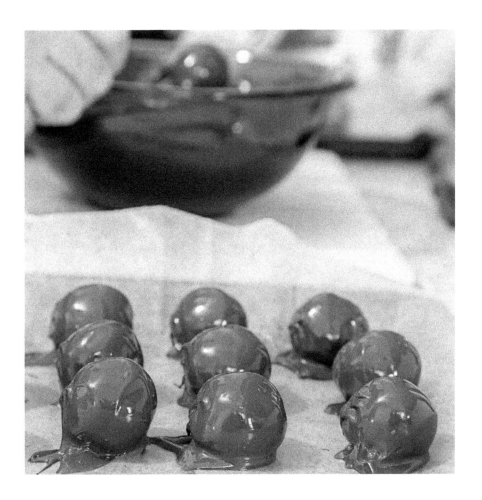

Other Keto Recipes

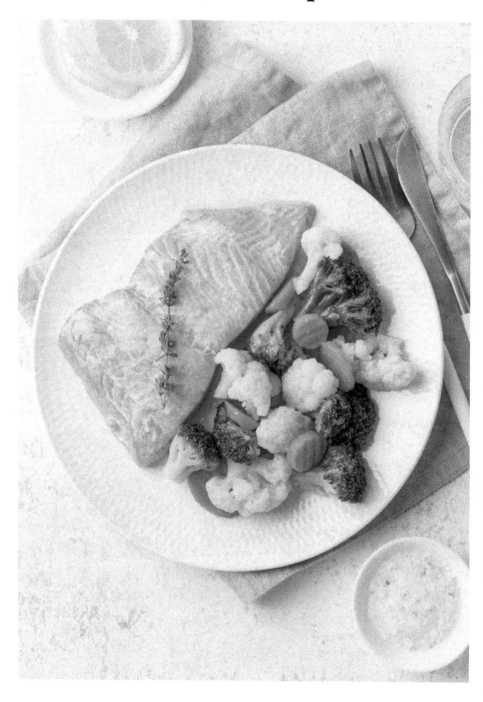

Omelette with Cabbage and Bacon

Preparation time: 7 minutes
Cooking time: 15 minutes
Servings: 4

Ingredients:
6 slices pancetta
4 tomatoes, cut into 1-inch chunks
1 large cucumber, seeded and sliced
1 small red onion, sliced
¼ cup balsamic vinegar
Salt and black pepper to taste
8 eggs
1 bunch kale, chopped
Salt and black pepper to taste
6 tablespoons grated Parmesan cheese
4 tablespoons olive oil
1 large white onion, sliced
3 ounces (85 g) beef salami, thinly sliced
1 clove garlic, minced

Directions:

Place the pancetta in a skillet and fry over medium heat until crispy, about 4 minutes. Remove to a cutting board and chop. Then, in a small bowl, whisk the vinegar, 2 tablespoons of olive oil, salt, and pepper to make the dressing. Next, combine the tomatoes, red onion, and cucumber in a salad bowl, drizzle with the dressing and toss the veggies. Sprinkle with the pancetta and set aside. Reheat the broiler to 400°F (205°C). Crack the eggs into a bowl and whisk together with half of the Parmesan, salt, and pepper. Set aside. Next, heat the remaining olive oil in the cast iron pan over medium heat. Sauté the onion and garlic for 3 minutes. Add the kale to the skillet, season with salt and pepper, and cook for 2 minutes. Top with the salami, stir and cook further for 1 minute. Pour the egg mixture all over the kale, reduce the heat to medium-low, cover, and cook the ingredients for 4 minutes. Sprinkle the remaining cheese on top and transfer the pan to the oven. Broil to brown on top for 1 minute. When ready, remove the pan and run a spatula around the edges of the frittata; slide it onto a warm platter. Cut the frittata into wedges and serve.

Nutrition:

calories: 454, fat: 30.1g, protein: 26.5g, carbs: 8.7g, net carbs: 4.5g, fiber: 4.2g

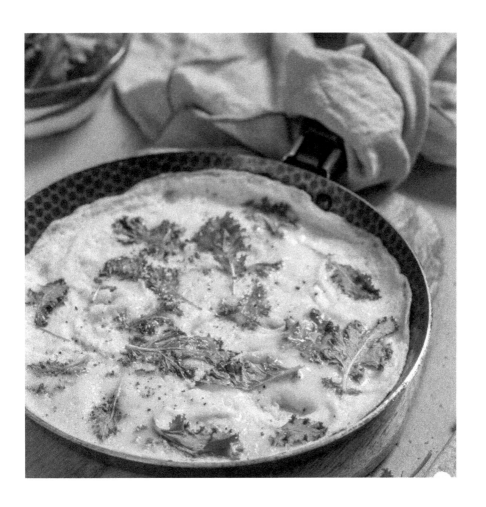

Chicken with Cheese

Preparation Time: 15 minutes
Cooking Time: 10 minutes
Servings: 6

Ingredients:
3 cups of chopped roasted chicken
2 cups of shredded cheddar cheese
cups white of shredded cheddar cheese
cups of shredded parmesan cheese

Directions:
Oven: 350F
Be sure to rub butter or to spray with non-stick cooking spray.
In a bowl, put in all the cheese and mix well.
Microwave the cheese till it melts
Put in the chicken and toss thoroughly.
Put two tablespoons of the cheese chicken combo in a pile on the baking sheet. Be sure to leave space between piles.
Bake for 4-6 minutes. The moment they turn golden brown at the edges, take them off.
Serve hot.

Nutrition:
calories 387, fat 19.5g, fiber 4.1g, carbohydrates 3.9 g, protein 14.5g

Stew with Sausage

Preparation time: 20 minutes
Cooking time: 30 minutes
Servings: 6

Ingredients:
1 pound (454 g) Italian sausage, sliced
red bell pepper, seeded and chopped
onions, chopped
Salt and black pepper, to taste
1 cup fresh parsley, chopped
6 green onions, chopped
¼ cup avocado oil
1 cup beef stock
4 garlic cloves
24 ounces (680 g) canned diced tomatoes
16 ounces (454 g) okra, trimmed and sliced
6 ounces (170 g) tomato sauce
2 tablespoons coconut aminos
1 tablespoon hot sauce

Directions:
Set a pot over medium heat and warm oil, place in the sausages, and
cook for 2 minutes. Stir in the onions, green onions, garlic, black
pepper, bell pepper, and salt, and cook for 5 minutes.
Add in the hot sauce, stock, tomatoes, coconut aminos, okra, and
tomato sauce, bring to a simmer and cook for 15 minutes. Adjust the
seasoning with salt and black pepper. Share into serving bowls and
sprinkle with fresh parsley to serve.

Nutrition:
calories 315, fat 25.1g, protein 16.1g, carbs 16.8g, net carbs 6.9g,
fiber 8.9g

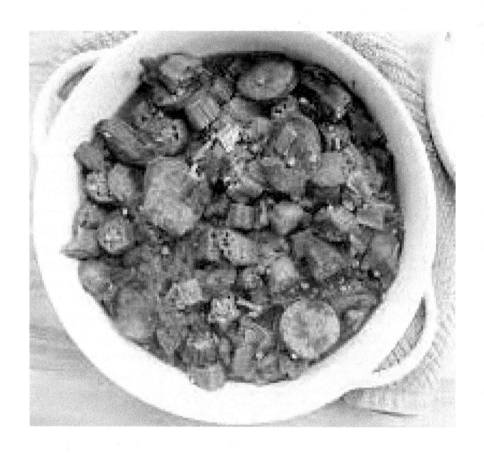

Crab Meatballs and Vegetables

Preparation time: 15 minutes
Cooking time: 10 minutes
ServIngs: 4

Ingredients:
1 large egg
¼ cup mayonnaise
1 green onion, chopped, plus extra for garnish (optional)
1 teaspoon Old Bay seasoning
1 tablespoon Dijon mustard
1 tablespoon chopped fresh parsley
1½ teaspoons fresh lemon juice
pound (454 g) fresh lump crabmeat
¼ cup golden flaxseed meal
to 3 tablespoons avocado oil, for frying
Spring mix greens or arugula, for serving (optional)
Lemon wedges, for serving (optional)

Directions:

In a large mixing bowl, combine the egg and mayonnaise and whisk until smooth. Add the green onion, Old Bay seasoning, mustard, parsley, and lemon juice and mix well. Sort through the crabmeat to ensure that no shells remain in the meat. Then add the crabmeat to the bowl with the egg mixture and gently mix with a spoon until well blended. Be sure to mix gently so that you don't break up the crabmeat too much. Gently fold in the flaxseed meal. Refrigerate the mixture for 20 to 30 minutes, then use your hands to form it into four 4-ounce (113-g) patties. Heat the avocado oil in a large skillet over medium-high heat. When hot, add the crab cakes and pan-fry for 4 to 5 minutes on each side, until golden brown and warm throughout. Serve immediately. If desired, serve each crab cake over a bed of spring mix or arugula with lemon wedges on the side and garnished with extra green onions.

Nutrition:

calories 333, fat 22.1g, protein 27.9g, carbs 3.7g, net carbs 1.8g, fiber: 1.9g

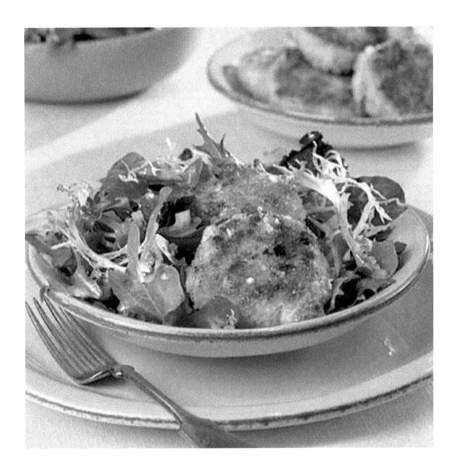

Beef and Spinach Salad

Preparation time: 15 minutes
Cooking time: 20 minutes
Servings: 4

Ingredients:
3 tablespoons olive oil
½ pound (227 g) beef rump steak, cut into strips
Salt and black pepper, to taste
1 teaspoon cumin
A pinch of dried thyme
2 garlic cloves, minced
4 ounces (113 g) Feta cheese, crumbled
½ cup pecans, toasted
2 cups spinach
1½ tablespoons lemon juice
¼ cup fresh mint, chopped

Directions:
Season the beef with salt, 1 tablespoon of olive oil, garlic, thyme, pepper, and cumin. Place on a preheated to medium heat grill, and cook for 10 minutes, flip once. Remove the grilled beef to a cutting board, leave to cool, and slice into strips.
Sprinkle the pecans on a lined baking sheet, place in the oven at 350°F (180°C), and toast for 10 minutes. In a salad bowl, combine the spinach with black pepper, mint, remaining olive oil, salt, lemon juice, Feta cheese, and pecans, and toss well to coat. Top with the beef slices and enjoy.

Nutrition:
calories 435, fat 43.1g, protein 17.1g, carbs 5.3g, net carbs 3.4g, fiber 1.9g

Balls with Sausage, Mortadella and Almonds

Preparation time: 15 minutes
Cooking time: 0 minutes
Servings: 4

Ingredients:
6 ounces (170 g) Mortadella sausage
6 bacon slices, cooked and crumbled
tablespoons almonds, chopped
½ teaspoon Dijon mustard
ounces (85 g) cream cheese

Directions:
Combine the mortadella and almonds in the bowl of your food processor.
Pulse until smooth. Whisk the cream cheese and mustard in another bowl.
Make balls out of the mortadella mixture. Make a thin cream cheese layer over.
Coat with bacon, arrange on a plate and chill before serving.

Nutrition:
calories 548, fat 51.2g, protein 21.6g, carbs 4.4g, net carbs 3.5g, fiber 0.9g

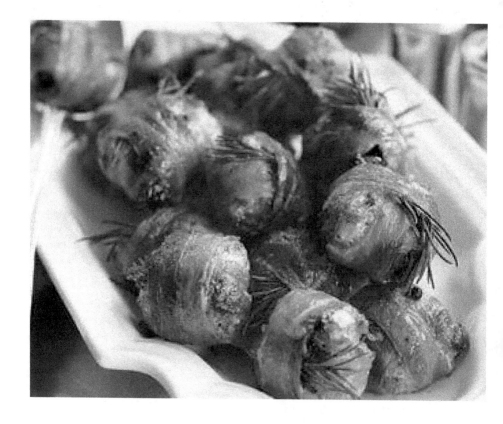

Turkey Soup with Green Beans

Preparation time: 20 minutes
Cooking time: 7 to 8 hours
Servings: 8

Ingredients:

1 tablespoon extra-virgin olive oil
4 cups chicken broth
½ pound (227 g) skinless turkey breast, cut into ½-inch chunks
2 celery stalks, chopped
1 carrot, diced
sweet onion, chopped
teaspoons minced garlic
2 teaspoons chopped fresh thyme
cup cream cheese, diced
cups heavy whipping cream
1 cup green beans, cut into 1-inch pieces
Salt, for seasoning

Directions:

Freshly ground black pepper, for seasoning
Lightly grease the insert of the slow cooker with the olive oil.
Place the broth, turkey, celery, carrot, onion, garlic, and thyme in the insert.
Cover and cook on low for 7 to 8 hours.
Stir in the cream cheese, heavy cream, and green beans.
Season with salt and pepper and serve.

Nutrition:

calories 416, fat 35.1g, protein 19.8g, carbs 7.0g, net carbs 5.0g, fiber 2.0g

Broccoli with Sardines

Preparation time: 5 minutes
Cooking time: 5 minutes
Servings: 4

Ingredients:
pound (454 g) broccoli florets
½ white onion, thinly sliced
(4-ounce / 113-g) cans sardines in oil, drained
2 tablespoons fresh lime juice
1 teaspoon stone-ground mustard

Directions:
Heat a lightly greased cast-iron skillet over medium-high heat. Cook the broccoli florets for 5 to 6 minutes until charred; work in batches.
In salad bowls, place the charred broccoli with onion and sardines. Toss with the lime juice and mustard. Serve at room temperature. Bon appétit!

Nutrition:
calories 160, fat 7.2g, protein 17.6g, carbs 5.6g, net carbs 2.6g, fiber 3.0g

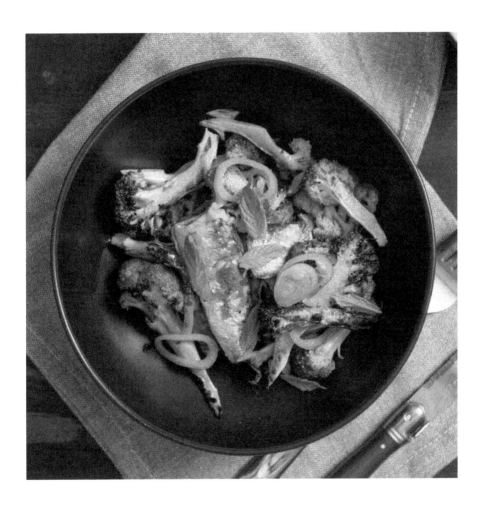

Mousse with Coffee and Chocolate

Preparation time: 10 minutes
Cooking time: 0 minutes
Servings: 6

Ingredients:

1 (13.5-ounce / 383-g) can coconut cream, chilled overnight
3 tablespoons granulated erythritol–monk fruit blend; less sweet: 2 tablespoons
2 tablespoons unsweetened cocoa powder, plus more for dusting
1 teaspoon instant espresso powder
¼ teaspoon salt

Directions:

Put the large metal bowl in the freezer to chill for at least 1 hour.
In the chilled large bowl, using an electric mixer on high, combine the coconut cream (adding it by the spoonful and reserving the water that has separated), erythritol–monk fruit blend, the cocoa powder, espresso powder, and salt and beat for 3 to 5 minutes, until stiff peaks form, stopping and scraping the bowl once or twice, as needed. If the consistency is too thick, add the reserved water from the coconut cream 1 tablespoon at a time to thin.
Serve immediately in a cold glass, dusted with cocoa powder.
Store leftovers in an airtight container for up to 5 days in the refrigerator.

Nutrition:

calories 126, fat 11.9g, protein 0g, carbs 3.1g, net carbs 2.0g, fiber 1.1g

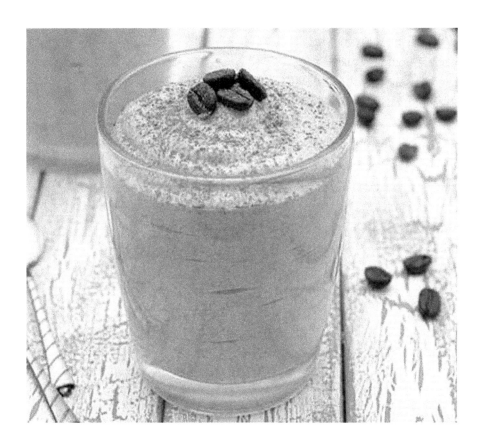

Sriracha Sauce

Preparation time: 5 minutes
Cooking time: 0 minutes
Makes: ¾ cup

Ingredients:
½ cup sugar-free mayonnaise
1½ tablespoons lime juice
1½ tablespoons Sriracha sauce
1 tablespoon granulated erythritol

Directions:
Place all of the ingredients in a small bowl and stir well until combined. Store in an airtight container in the refrigerator for up to 1 week.

Nutrition:
calories 140, fat 15.8g, protein 0g, carbs 1.0g, net carbs 1.0g, fiber 0g

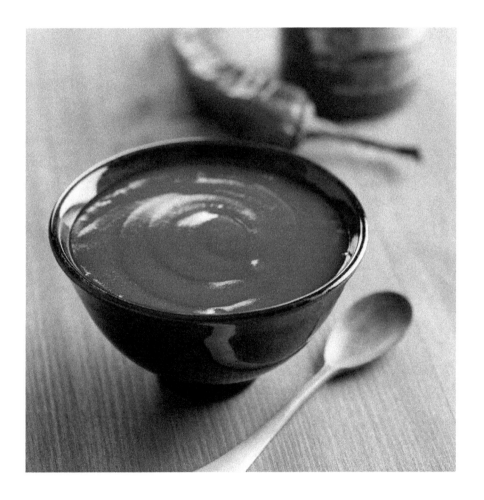

CPSIA information can be obtained
at www.ICGtesting.com
Printed in the USA
LVHW051134110621
689903LV00005B/485